AIR FRYER BASICS COOKBOOK

and

AIR FRYER HEALTHY COOKBOOK

2 in 1 Bundle:

Easy and Delicious Healthy Recipes,
Finally Enjoy your Favorite Fried
Foods Without Thinking About the Fat
Content.
Crispy Goodness to Prepare for You,
Family and Friends.

Violet H.Scott

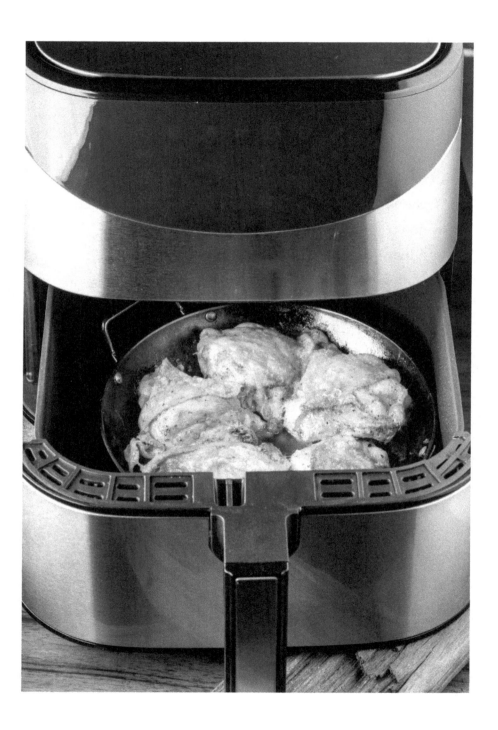

Table of Contents

Air Fryer Basic Cookbook

Introduction.. **8**

Air fryer, what is it?.. 10

How does the oil-free hot air fryer work? 11

Your advantages with a hot air fryer...................................... 12

A few numbers about air fryers.. 13

AIR FRYER MUSHROOMS 14

WHOLE GRILLED CHICKEN.................................15

AIR FRYER LIGHT ASPARAGUS 18

KETO ZUCCHINI FRIES......................................20

YUMMY SLICED BACON....................................23

AIR FRYER POTATOES CHIPS 24

AIR FRYER ONION RINGS 26

YUMMY BACON-WRAPPED DATES 29

TASTY BACON-WRAPPED SHRIMP 30

AIR FRYER CHILI SHRIMP 32

TASTY SWEET POTATO TOAST 35

AIR FRYER KALE CHIPS....................................36

ROASTED BELL PEPPERS 38

AIR-FRIED BROCCOLI CRISPS............................40

CRISPY KETO CROUTONS 42

TASTY APPLE CHEESE 44

YUMMY AND CHEESY HASH BROWN BRUSCHETTA ...46

PAPRIKA PORK CHOPS.. 48

EGGPLANT SIDE DISH 50

SANDWICHES NUTS & CHEESE 52

AIR FRYER BROCCOLI..54

AIR FRYER JALAPEÑO BURGER BITES 56

HEALTHY PARMESAN BRUSSEL SPROUTS....................59

AIR FRYER CHICKEN THIGHS 62

CHICKPEA & CARROT BALLS 65

SUCCULENT CHICKEN NUGGETS FOR AIR FRYER 66

LIGHT CHICKEN AND VEGETABLES WITH AIR FRYER
.... 68

EXQUISITE VEGETABLES BROWNED WITH THE AIR
FRYER 70

CHICKPEA & CARROT BALLS 73

TASTY AIR FRYER MOZZARELLA STICKS.......................75

CRISPY AND SOFT JALAPENO POPPERS BALLS............78

EASY AIR FRYER TUNA STEAKS 82

AIR FRYER LEMON SHRIMP 84

DELICIOUS AIR FRYER BACON-WRAPPED STUFFED
JALAPENOS..87

KETO AIR FRYER GARLIC CHICKEN BREAST.............. 90

RIBEYE STEAK FRIES 93

AIR FRYER LEMON COD LOINS 96

AIR FRYER CHICKEN FAJITAS......................................99

SAUSAGE BREAKFAST PATTIES 102

AIR FRYER SALMON FILLETS 104

AIR FRIED CHICKEN DRUMSTICKS BBQ SAUCE 107

Conclusion 110

Air Fryer Healthy Cookbook

Introduction 114
Air fryer recipes 116

PAPRIKA POTATO FRIES 116
OVEN ZUCCHINI WITH SMOKED SALMON 118
AIR FRYER HALLOUMI 120
LOW CARB SALMON CAKES 122
DELICIOUS POTATO CAULIFLOWER PATTIES............ 126
AIR FRYER ITALIAN ZUCCHINI CHIPS....................... 129
AIR FRYER JUMBO SHRIMP 132
LOW CARB RANCH STEAK NUGGETS........................ 134
AIR FRYER SALMON FILLETS TERIYAKI 137
AIR FRYER AVOCADO 140
Creamy Chicken, Rice, And Peas 143
AIR FRYER KETO QUESO FUNDIDO 144
AIR FRYER TILAPIA FILLETS 146
AIR FRYER FLANK STEAK WITH CHIMICHURRI SAUCE
.... 148
AIR FRYER SCALLOPS WITH TOMATO CREAM SAUCE
.... 150
CRISPY AIR FRYER BRUSSELS SPROUTS 152
AIR FRYER VEGETABLE CHIPS 154
AIR FRYER CINNAMON QUARK BALLS 156

OVEN GREEN CURRY DRUMSTICKS 158

AIR FRYER VEGAN CHICKEN WINGS 160

AIR FRYER BROCCOLI 163

AIR FRYER BLISSFUL SALMON 165

AIR FRYER BROCCOLI 168

AIR FRYER CAULIFLOWER CROQUETTES!.................. 170

AIR FRYER CRISPY TOFU.. 172

AIR FRYER BEEF KOFTA KABAB 174

AIRFRYER HEALTHY SANDWICH 176

VEGETABLE PAPRIKA CHIPS 178

ZUCCHINI AND CHEESE BREAD 180

LOW CARB PARMESAN BREAD................................. 182

AIRFRYER CINNAMON CARROT CAKE....................... 184

AIR FRYER ALMOND CHICKEN 186

DUCK BREAST SAUCE 189

TASTY CRISPY CHICKEN BREASTS............................ 190

PAPRIKA CHICKEN TENDERS.................................... 192

CHICKEN THIGHS WITH PEANUTS 193

SIMPLE CHICKEN THIGHS.. 194

BBQ CHICKEN WINGS 195

ORANGE JUICE MARINATED STEAK 196

Conclusion 198

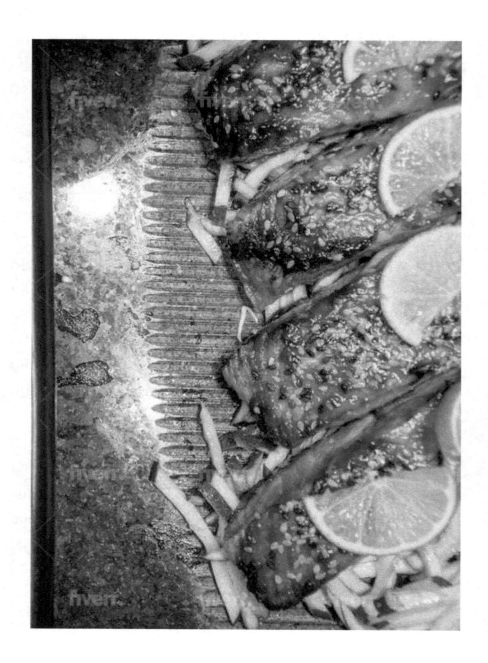

8

AIR FRYER BASICS COOKBOOK

Easy and Delicious Recipes On a Budget for Quick and Easy Meals. From Crispy Fries and Juicy Steaks to Perfect Veggies, What and How to Cook for the Best Results
Including Low-Carb Recipes That Will Help You Stay Healthy and Lose Weight.

Violet H.Scott

Introduction

Air fryer, what is it?

The air fryer is basically an upgraded tabletop ventilation oven. This small device aims to achieve frying results with only hot air and very little or no oil.

This device has become very popular in recent years - about 45% of US homes have one. There are all kinds of things you can air-fry, from frozen chicken wings to French fries, from roasted vegetables to freshly baked cookies.

It allows you to cook food within a stream of hot air. In this process, the food is spun in this stream of air and then fried. Compared to traditional fryers, there is no need for much fat. Today's technology allows for the preparation of delicacies that retain their natural taste.

How does the oil-free hot air fryer work?

Inside the hot air fryer is a heating ring that allows the air to rise to a temperature of 40 to 200 degrees. The hot air is then distributed into the oven by a fan. Compared to the oven, the speed of hot air circulation is more consistent. This ensures that the dishes are as crispy as with the classic fryer. The cooking is faster, which saves on energy costs. However, its noise during use is high. With an average of 75 dB, the hot air fryer is almost as loud as a regular hair dryer or vacuum cleaner.

With the hot air fryer, you can not only fry food but also heat; for example vegetables, you can bake cakes or grill meat.

Your advantages with a hot air fryer

- tasty and healthy food
- vitamin-rich food
- low-fat preparation of food
- natural taste is retained
- quick and easy cleaning thanks to the easy-care production method
- Can be used in many ways: baking, roasting, grilling, cooking, defrosting, deep-frying
- no grease odor in the house, no grease stains
- easily usable for diabetics and dieters
- Food does not lose moisture
- ideal for private individuals and (large) families
- safe and easy application
- Fry French fries with 80 percent less fat
- Food rotates in a stream of hot air and does not swim in hot fat
- Preparation of fish, meat and vegetables

A few numbers about air fryers

The body derives numerous benefits from the use of this product.

The preparation of fries requires 80 percent less fat than a regular fryer.

French fries made from fresh potatoes contain about three percent fat, those from conventional fryers up to 20 percent. Frozen fries cooked with hot air, on the other hand, have only about six percent fat. A serving of conventional fries (about 250 grams) has just under 700 calories, while hot air fries have only 500. That's why its use is becoming increasingly popular.

AIR FRYER MUSHROOMS

Yield: 2 servings

Prep time: 10 mins Cook time: 15 mins Total time: 25 mins

Ingredients

8 oz. (227 g) mushrooms, washed and dried

1-2 Tablespoons (15-30 ml) olive oil

1/2 teaspoon (2.5 ml) garlic powder

1 teaspoon (5 ml) Worcestershire or soy sauce

Kosher salt, to taste

black pepper, to taste

lemon wedges (optional)

1 Tablespoon (15 ml) chopped parsley

Instructions

Make sure mushrooms are evenly cut for even cooking. Cut mushrooms in half or quarters (depending on preferred size).

Add to bowl then toss with oil, garlic powder, Worcestershire/soy sauce, salt and pepper

Air fry at 380°F for 10-12 minutes, tossing and shaking half way through. Adjust cooking time to your preferred doneness.

Drizzle and squeeze some fresh lemon juice and top with chopped parsley. Serve warm. Yum!

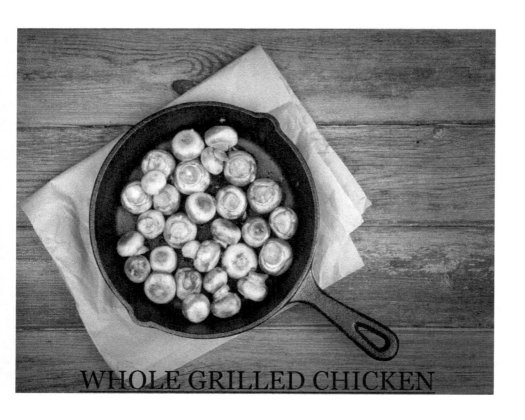

WHOLE GRILLED CHICKEN

Servings 3-4,

Preparation: 5 min

 Cooking time 30-40 min

Ingredients

1 whole chicken (about 800 g)

2 tablespoons olive oil

Salt

Pepper

Fresh thyme

1 whole garlic

1 lemon

Instructions

Rinse the chicken in cold water and pat it dry with kitchen paper.

2. Then brush or rub the oil over the whole chicken.

3. Salt and pepper

4. Place the thyme sprigs in the bottom of the Air fryer basket, and place the chicken on top.

5. Divide the lemon in half and rub the juice of one half over the chicken, and place the other half in the basket next to the chicken.

Divide the garlic in half and place them in the basket together with the chicken.

Cook in the Air fryer at 180 ° C, 30-40 minutes.

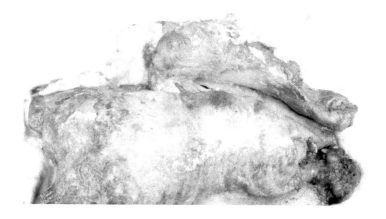

AIR FRYER LIGHT ASPARAGUS

Prep Time: 4 minutes Cook Time: 7 minutes

Servings: 4 Calories: 55kcal

Ingredients

1 lb asparagus

1/4 tsp salt

1/8 tsp black pepper

1 Tbsp avocado oil

1 garlic clove pressed

Instructions

Start by snapping off the end of each asparagus spare. The ends tend to be quite chewy so you want to get rid of them. You want to remove about 1 to 2 inches from the bottom.

Now place the trimmed asparagus on a rimmed baking sheet and drizzle with avocado oil. Then mix in the pressed or grated garlic clove.

Now season with salt and pepper and toss them until they are well coated in the seasoning.

Place the seasoned asparagus on the air fryer basket and cook on high (450 degrees) for 7 minutes.

Enjoy!

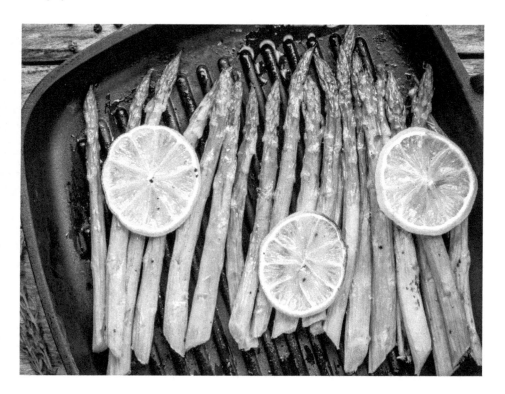

KETO ZUCCHINI FRIES

yield: 6 SERVINGS prep time: 15 MINUTES cook time: 25 MINUTES total time: 40 MINUTE

Ingredients

2 medium zucchini

1 egg

1/4 tsp salt

1 cup almond flour

1/2 cup grated Parmesan cheese

1 tsp garlic powder

1 tsp Italian herb blend

Instructions

Preheat the oven to 425 degrees Fahrenheit and line a large baking sheet with parchment paper.

Slice the zucchini in half crosswise. Then, cut again lengthwise into sticks.

Crack the egg in a shallow bowl and lightly beat it with the salt.

Add the almond flour, parmesan, garlic, and herbs to a separate shallow bowl and stir to combine.

Using one hand, dip a piece of zucchini in the egg wash, let excess egg drip off, and transfer to the almond/parmesan mixture. Using your other hand, press the zucchini in the almond/parmesan mixture to coat. Place on the baking sheet in a single layer. Repeat this process until all zucchini pieces are coated. Spray with olive oil.

Bake for 25-30 minutes, flipping halfway through. Serve immediately.

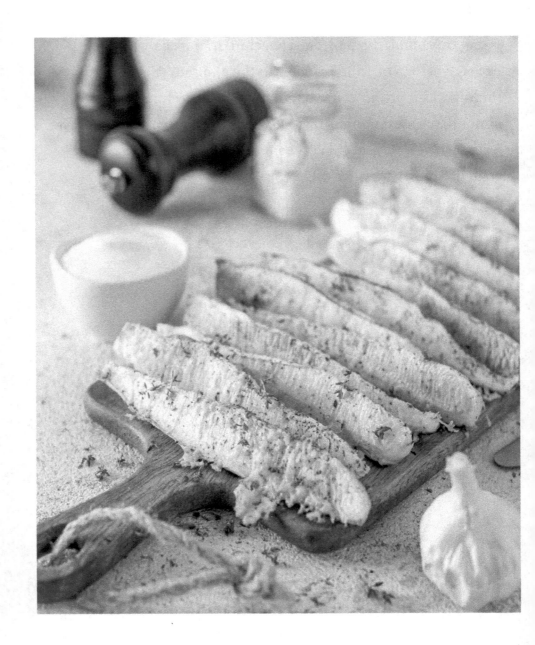

YUMMY SLICED BACON

Cooking Time: 10 min

Servings: 2

Ingredients

•Brown sugar - 3 tbsp.

•Water - 2 tbsp.

•Eight slices bacon

•Maple syrup - 2 tbsp.

Instructions

First adjust the air fryer to heat at 400°F. Remove the basket and cover the base with baking paper.

Then empty the water into the base of the fryer while preheating.

In a glass dish add and whisk the 2 tbsp. Of maple syrup and the 3 tbsp. Brown sugar together.

Place the wire rack into the basket and arrange the bacon into a single layer.

After that spread the sugar glaze on the bacon until completely covered.

Then put the basket into the air fryer and steam for 8 minutes.

Then move the bacon from the basket and wait about 5 minutes before serving hot.

AIR FRYER POTATOES CHIPS

Prep Time

15 mins

Cook Time

25 mins

Total Time

40 mins

Ingredients

4 medium yellow potatoes

1 tbsp oil

salt to taste

Instructions

Slice the potatoes into thin slices. Place them into a bowl with cold water and let it soak for at least 20 minutes.

Remove from water, pat dry with a towel.

Season the potato chips with salt and oil. Place them in an air fryer and cook for 20 minutes at 200°F.

Toss the potato chips, turn up heat to 400°F and cook for about 5 more minutes

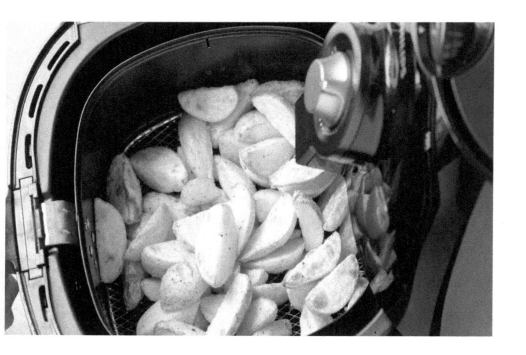

AIR FRYER ONION RINGS

Prep Time

20 mins

Cook Time

10 mins

Total Time

30 mins

Servings: 6

Ingredients

1 large sweet onion cut into rings

1 cup almond flour

1 cup grated Parmesan cheese

1 tablespoon baking powder

1 teaspoon smoked paprika

Salt and pepper

2 eggs beaten

1 tablespoon heavy cream

cooking spray

Instructions

In a medium bowl, combine the almond flour, Parmesan cheese, baking powder, smoked paprika, salt, and pepper.

Beat the eggs and heavy cream in another bowl.

Dip the onion rings in the eggs and then in the almond flour mixture. Press the almond flour mixture into the onions. Transfer to a parchment lined baking sheet and repeat with the remaining onion.

Air Fryer Instructions

Preheat your air fryer to 350 degrees. Arrange the onions in a single layer, cooking in batches as needed. (If desired, you can line your air fryer with air fryer liners.)

Spray the onions with cooking spray and cook for 5 minutes. Use a spatula to carefully reach under the onions and flip. Respray and cook 5 minutes longer.

Baking Instructions

Preheat the oven to 400 degrees. Line a baking sheet with parchment paper. Arrange the onions in a single layer and spray with cooking spray. Bake for 10 minutes. Flip and respray with oil. Bake another 10 to 12 minutes, until crispy and brown.

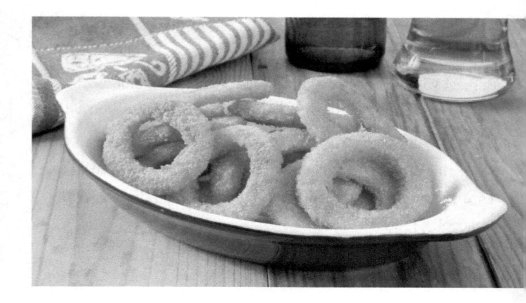

YUMMY BACON-WRAPPED DATES

Cooking Time: 6 min Servings: 6

Ingredients:

•12 dates, pitted

•Six slices of high-quality bacon, cut in half

•Cooking spray

Instructions

Start by preheating the air fryer oven to 360°F (182°C).

Then use half a bacon slice to wrap each date and secure it with a toothpick.

Spritz the air fryer basket using cooking spray, and then place bacon- wrapped dates in the basket.

Put the air fryer basket and the select Air Fry, and set the time to 6 minutes, or until the bacon is crispy.

Remove the dates and allow cooling on a wire rack for 5 minutes before serving.

TASTY BACON-WRAPPED SHRIMP

Cooking Time: 13 min Servings: 8

Ingredients:

- 24 large shrimp, peeled and deveined, about ¾ pound (340 g)
- Five tbsps. barbecue sauce, divided
- 12 strips bacon, cut in half
- 24 small pickled jalapeño slices

Instructions

First you need to toss together the shrimp and 3 tbsps. Of the barbecue sauce. Let stand for 15 minutes. Soak 24 wooden toothpicks in water for 10 minutes. Wrap one piece of bacon around the shrimp and jalapeño slice, then secure with a toothpick.

Start by preheating the air fryer oven, set the temperature to 350°F (177°C).

Then place the shrimp in the air fryer basket, spacing them ½ inch apart, select Air Fry, and set time to 10 minutes.

Turn shrimp over with tongs and air fry for 3 minutes more, or until bacon is golden brown and shrimp are cooked through.

Brush with the remaining barbecue sauce and serve.

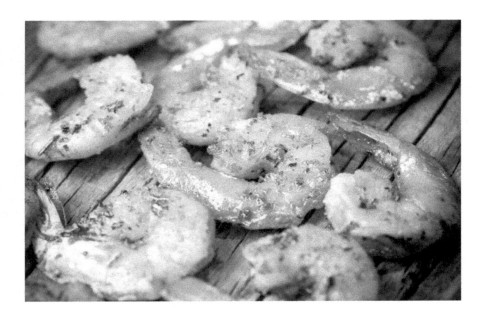

AIR FRYER CHILI SHRIMP

Prep Time

10 mins

Cook Time

12 mins

0 mins

Total Time

22 mins

Servings: 4 servings

Ingredients

1 pound shrimp raw, large, peeled and deveined with tails attached

¼ cup all-purpose flour

½ teaspoon salt

¼ teaspoon black pepper

2 large eggs

¾ cup unsweetened shredded coconut

¼ cup panko breadcrumbs

Cooking spray

Sweet chili sauce for serving

Instructions

Preheat the air fryer to 360°F. When heated, spray the basket with cooking spray.

Combine the flour, salt and pepper in one shallow bowl. Whisk the eggs in a second shallow bowl. Then combine the shredded coconut and panko breadcrumbs in a third shallow bowl.

Dip the shrimp into the flour mixture, shaking off any excess. Then dredge the shrimp into the eggs, and finally into the coconut panko mixture, gently pressing to adhere.

Place the coconut shrimp in the air fryer so they are not touching, and spray the top of the shrimp. Cook for 10-12 minutes, flipping halfway through.

Garnish with chopped parsley, and serve immediately with sweet chili sauce, if desired.

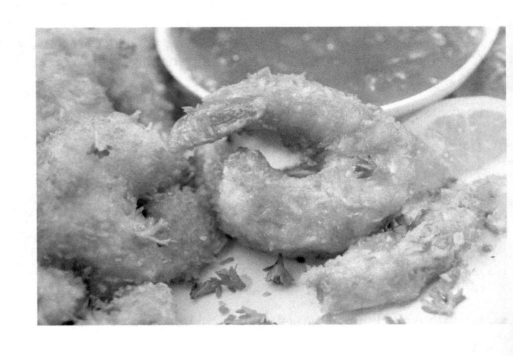

TASTY SWEET POTATO TOAST

Cooking Time:30 Min   Servings:2

Ingredients

•Salt - 1/4 tsp.

•Paprika seasoning - 1/8 tsp.

•Avocado oil - 4 tsp.

•Garlic powder - 1/8 tsp.

•Onion powder - 1/8 tsp.

•Pepper - 1/4 tsp.

•Oregano seasoning - 1/8 tsp.

•One sweet potato

Instructions

Start by heating the air fryer to the temperature of 380°F.

Then cut the ends off the sweet potato and discard. Divide into four even pieces lengthwise.

And whisk the avocado oil and all of the seasonings until combined thoroughly.

Brush the spices on top of the slices of sweet potato.

After that transfer the slices to the air fryer basket and fry for 15 minutes.

Turn the sweet potato pieces over and steam once again for 15 more minutes.

Remove to a serving plate and enhance with your preferred toppings.

AIR FRYER KALE CHIPS

prep time: 5 MINUTES cook time: 7 MINUTES total time: 12 MINUTES

ingredients

1 batch curly kale, washed and patted dry

2 teaspoons olive oil

1 tablespoon nutritional yeast

¼ teaspoon sea salt

1/8 teaspoon ground black pepper

instructions

Remove the leaves from the stems of the kale and place them in a medium bowl.

Add the olive oil, nutritional yeast, salt, and pepper. Use your hands to massage the toppings into the kale leaves.

Pour the kale into the basket of your air fryer and cook on 390 degrees F for 6-7 minutes, or until they are crispy.

Serve warm or at room temperature.

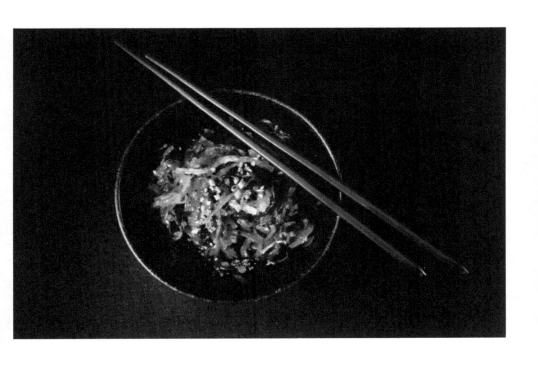

ROASTED BELL PEPPERS

Preparation Time: 8 minutes Cooking Time: 22 minutes
Servings: 4

Ingredients:

One red bell pepper

One yellow bell pepper

One orange bell pepper

One green bell pepper

2 tbsps. olive oil, divided

½ tsp. dried marjoram

Pinch salt

Freshly ground black pepper

One head garlic

Instructions

Slice the bell peppers into 1-inch strips.

In a prepared large bowl, toss the bell peppers with 1 tbsp of the oil. Sprinkle on the marjoram, salt, and pepper, and toss again.

Trim the top of the head of the garlic and place the cloves on an oiled square of aluminum foil. Drizzle with the remaining olive oil. Wrap the garlic in the foil.

Place the wrapped garlic in the air fryer and roast for 15 minutes, then add the bell peppers. Roast for 7 minutes or until the peppers are tender and the garlic is soft. Transfer the peppers to a serving dish.

Remove the garlic from the air fryer and unwrap the foil. When cool enough to handle, squeeze the garlic cloves out of the papery skin and mix with the bell peppers.

Cooking tip: To easily remove the seeds from a dash of bell pepper, cut around the stem with a sharp knife and simply pull out the stem with the seeds attached. Rinse the pepper to remove any stray seeds and cut them into strips.

AIR-FRIED BROCCOLI CRISPS

Preparation Time: 10 minutes

Cooking Time: 12 minutes

Servings: 4

Ingredients

One large broccoli head, chopped

2 tbsps. olive oil

1 tsp. black pepper

1 tsp. salt

Instructions:

Set your Air Fryer Oven temperature to 360 degrees F

Take a bowl and add broccoli florets, olive oil, salt, and black pepper

Then toss them well

Add the broccoli florets

Cook for 12 minutes

Shake after 6 minutes

Remove it from your air fryer and let it cool before serve

Serve and enjoy!

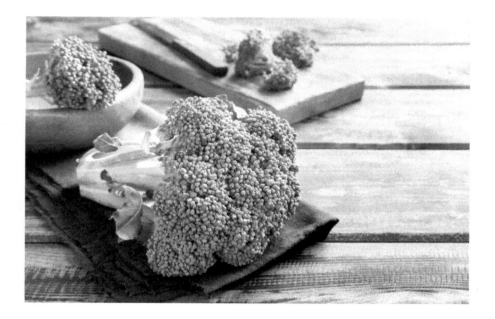

CRISPY KETO CROUTONS

Prep time10 minutes Cook time10 minutes Total time 20 minutes

Ingredients

2 Cups of Keto Farmers Bread (200g) half of the loaf

1 Tbsp of Marjoram

2Tbsp Olive Oil

1/2 Tbsp Garlic Powder

Instructions

As I have already mentioned our Keto Farmers Bread is used in this recipe.

Make sure your bread is cooled. Cut it into same size slices and then squares.

Place all of the croutons into a big bowl, which would be spacious enough to mix all the herbs and oil.

Add oil, Dry Garlic and Marjoram.

With a big spatula, mix all of the croutons fully. Do not forget to make sure the oil and herbs are spread evenly.

Depending on your Air Fryer, fill it up with your Keto Croutons. Make sure you only add one layer, otherwise they will not crisp fully.

Switch the Air Fryer on. You do not need to add additional oil, since you have already coated your Keto Croutons with oil before.

After 10 minutes the Crunchy Keto Croutons are ready to be served. Let them cool or serve them still hot or warm. It all depends for what you want to use them.

Bon Appetit

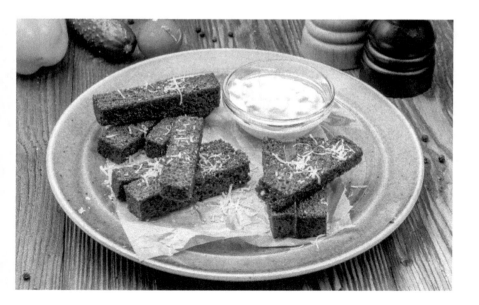

TASTY APPLE CHEESE

Cooking Time: 5 min Servings: 8 roll-ups

Ingredients:

Eight slices whole wheat sandwich bread

4 ounces (113 g) Colby Jack cheese, grated

½ small apple, chopped

2 tbsps. butter, melted

Instructions

Start by preheating the air fryer oven to 390°F (199°C).

Take the crusts from the bread and flatten the slices with a rolling pin. Don't be gentle. Press hard so that the bread will be very thin.

Then top the bread slices with cheese and chopped apple, dividing the ingredients evenly.

After that roll up each slice tightly and secure each with one or two toothpicks.

Brush outside of rolls with melted butter. Place them in the air fryer basket.

Putting the air fryer basket onto the baking pan and select Air Fry, and set time to 5 minutes, or until outside is crisp and nicely browned.

Serve hot.

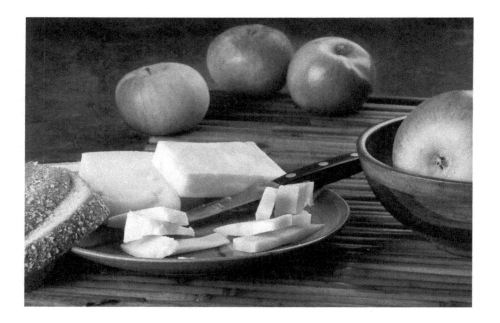

YUMMY AND CHEESY HASH BROWN BRUSCHETTA

Cooking Time: 8 min Servings: 4

Ingredients:

Four frozen hash brown patties

1 tbsp. olive oil

1/3 cup chopped cherry tomatoes

3 tbsps. diced fresh Mozzarella

2 tbsps. grated Parmesan cheese

1 tbsp. balsamic vinegar

1 tbsp. minced fresh basil

Instructions

Start by preheating the air fryer oven temperature to 400°F (204°C).

Put the hash brown patties in the air fryer basket in a single layer.

Then put the air fryer basket onto the baking pan and select Air Fry, set time to 8 minutes, or wait until the potatoes are crisp, hot, and golden brown.

In the meantime and combine the olive oil, tomatoes, Mozzarella, Parmesan, vinegar, and basil in a small bowl.

When the potatoes are finished, you can remove them from the basket carefully and arrange them on a serving plate. Top with the tomato mixture and serve.

PAPRIKA PORK CHOPS

Prep Time 5 minutes

Cook Time 12 minutes

Servings 4

Ingredients

8 oz pork chops (four) bone-in center-cut, or boneless (see recipe notes)

1 tsp olive oil

Pork Chop Seasoning

1 tsp paprika

1 tsp onion powder

1 tsp salt

1 tsp pepper

instructions

Preheat your air fryer to 380°F.

Brush both sides of pork chop with a little olive oil.

Mix the pork seasonings together in a bowl (this is enough for four pork chops) and apply to both sides of the pork chop.

Place pork chop in air fryer and cook for between 9-12 minutes, turning the chop over halfway, until it reaches a minimum temp of 145°F (exact cook time will vary depending on thickness of pork and your model of air fryer)

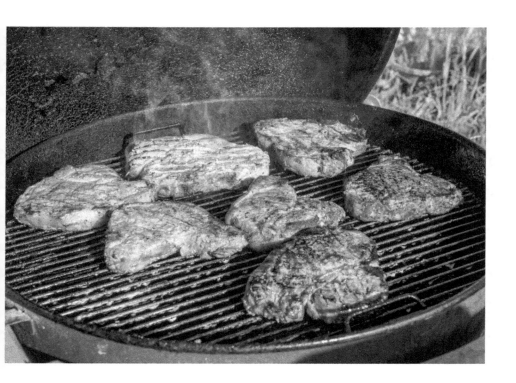

EGGPLANT SIDE DISH

Preparation Time: 10 minutes Cooking Time: 10 minutes
Servings: 4

Ingredients

Eight baby eggplants

½ tsp. garlic powder

One yellow onion, chopped

One green bell pepper, chopped

One bunch coriander, chopped

1 tbsp. tomato paste

1 tbsp. olive oil

One tomato, chopped

Salt and black pepper

Instructions

Place a pan over heat and then add the oil.

Melt the oil and fry the onion for 1 minute

Add green bell pepper, oregano, eggplant pulp, tomato, coriander, garlic powder, tomato paste, salt, and pepper. Stir-fry for 2 minutes

Remove from the heat and let it cool

Arrange them in your Air fryer

Cook for 8 minutes at 360 degrees F

Serve and enjoy!

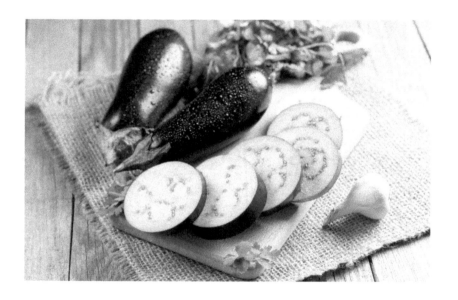

SANDWICHES NUTS & CHEESE

Preparation Time: 10 minutes Cooking Time: 50 minutes
Servings: 2

Ingredients

One heirloom tomato

1 (4-oz) block feta cheese

One small red onion, thinly sliced

One clove garlic

Salt to taste

2 tsp. + ¼ cup olive oil

1 ½ tbsp. toasted pine nuts

¼ cup chopped parsley

¼ cup grated Parmesan cheese

¼ cup chopped basil

Instructions

Add basil, pine nuts, garlic, and salt to a food processor. Process while slowly adding ¼ cup of olive oil. Once finished, pour basil pesto into a bowl and refrigerate for 30 minutes.

Preheat on Air Fry function to 390 F. Slice the feta cheese and tomato into ½-inch slices. Remove the pesto from the fridge and spread half of it on the tomato slices. Top with feta cheese slices and onion. Drizzle the remaining olive oil on top.

Place the tomatoes in the fryer basket and fit in the baking tray; cook for 12 minutes. Remove to a serving platter and top with the remaining pesto. Serve.

AIR FRYER BROCCOLI

Prep time 5 minutes

Cook time 6 minutes

Total time 11 minutes

Yield: 4 servings

Ingredients

1 head of broccoli

2 tablespoons butter, melted

1 clove garlic, minced

salt and pepper to taste

1/4 cup Parmesan cheese (freshly grated)

additional parmesan cheese for serving

pinch of red pepper flakes (optional)

Instructions

Preheat your air fryer to 400 degrees.

Cut broccoli into florets and set aside.

Mix together melted butter, minced garlic, salt, pepper, and red pepper flakes (if using).

Add the broccoli and mix to combine thoroughly.

Add the Parmesan cheese and mix again making sure to coat it evenly.

Place broccoli into the air fryer and cook for 6-8 minutes, shaking the basket halfway through. *

Remove broccoli from the air fryer and serve immediately.

Add additional Parmesan cheese on top once served.

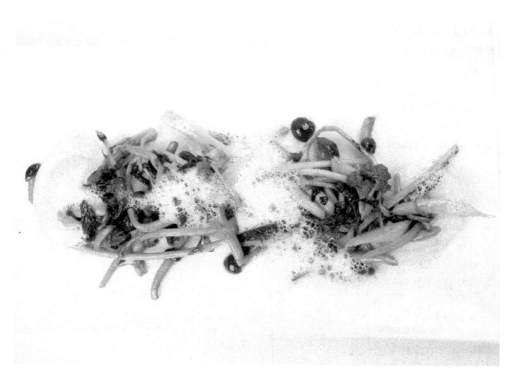

AIR FRYER JALAPEÑO BURGER BITES

PREP TIME:

10 mins

COOK TIME:

20 mins

TOTAL TIME:

30 mins

YIELD:15 SERVINGS

Ingredients

2 lbs. 90% beef

4 oz center cut raw bacon, minced

2 tablespoons yellow mustard

1/2 tsp kosher salt

1/2 tsp onion powder

1/4 tsp black pepper

1 head butter lettuce

30 cherry tomatoes

2-3 jalapeño sliced in 30 thin slices, optional

30 dill pickle chips or slices

ketchup, mayo and/or yellow mustard, optional for dipping

Instructions

Using your hands, gently mix together the beef, bacon, mustard, salt, onion powder and pepper.

Form into 30 (golf ball size) balls.

Preheat the air fryer 400F. Working in batches arrange burgers in a single layer.

Cook, flipping halfway to your desired doneness, 8 to 10 minutes for medium.

Place each burger on a skewer with lettuce, pickles and tomatoes and serve with dipping sauces.

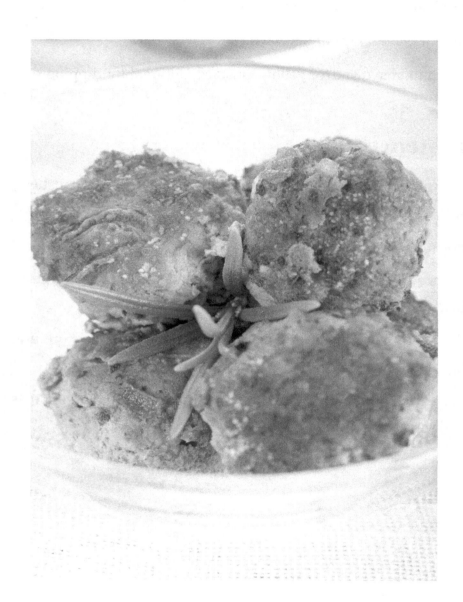

HEALTHY PARMESAN BRUSSEL SPROUTS

Prep Time

10 mins

Cook Time

12 mins

25

Servings: 4 serves

Ingredients

1 pound Brussel Sprouts, ends trimmed, outer leaves removed, and cut in half, lengthwise

1 tablespoon olive oil

1/2 teaspoon garlic powder

1/4 teaspoon salt

1/8 teaspoon ground black pepper

1/4 cup pork panko bread crumbs

1/4 cup grated Parmesan cheese

Instructions

In a large bowl combine prepared Brussel sprouts, olive oil, garlic powder, salt, and pepper; stir until thoroughly incorporated.

Transfer Brussel sprouts to the air fryer's basket and cook for 6 minutes at 400°F.

When time is up, open the air fryer, stir around the Brussel sprouts.

Sprinkle sprouts with parmesan cheese and pork panko crumbs.

Arrange in one layer and continue to air fry for an additional 5 to 7 minutes, or until crisp tender.

Remove sprouts from air fryer.

Test for seasonings and adjust accordingly.

Serve.

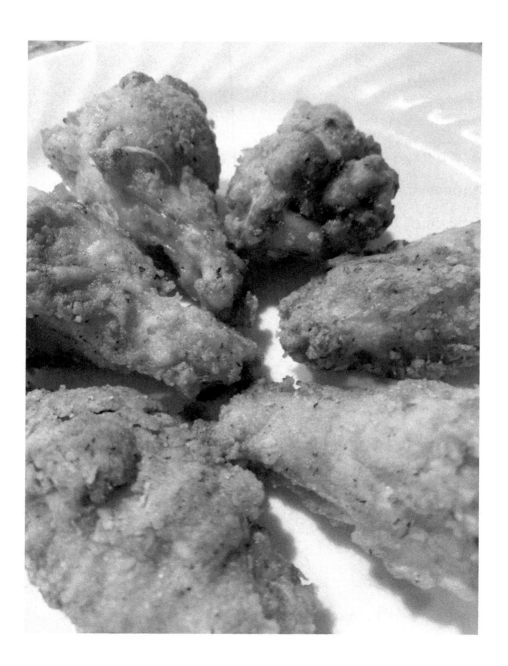

AIR FRYER CHICKEN THIGHS

Prep time 10 mins

Cook time 25 mins

Marinate time 1 hr.

Total time 1 hr. 35 mins

Servings 4 servings

Ingredients

1.5 lbs. boneless skinless chicken thighs

1/3 cup soy sauce

3 Tb Swerve brown sugar or brown sugar if not keto

1/2 tsp ginger paste

1/2 tsp garlic powder

1/4 tsp onion powder

1/4 tsp black pepper

2-3 Tb green onions chopped for garnish

1-2 tsp sesame seeds for garnish

Instructions

To a small bowl, whisk together the soy sauce, swerve brown sugar substitute (or regular brown sugar if don't want to keep this recipe keto), ginger paste, garlic powder, onion powder, and black pepper.

Pour the marinade into a zip top bag and add the chicken. Seal the bag then toss to coat well.

Let the chicken marinate in the fridge for at least one hour, but up to overnight.

Preheat your air fryer to 350 degrees.

Cook the chicken on a rack in the air fryer for 20-25 minutes until nicely browned and cooked through.

Let rest in the air fryer with the heat off for a few minutes.

Garnish with chopped green onions and sesame seeds before serving.

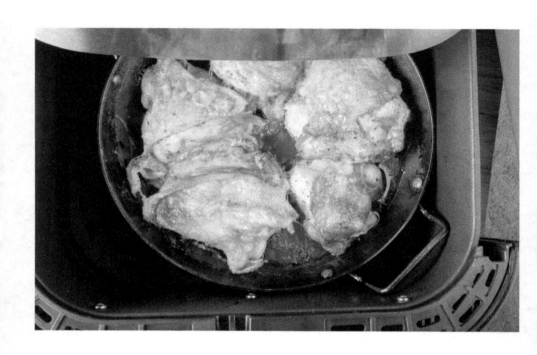

CHICKPEA & CARROT BALLS

Preparation Time: 5 minutes Cooking Time: 20 minutes
Servings: 3

Ingredients

2 tbsp. olive oil

2 tbsp. soy sauce

1 tbsp. flax meal

2 cups cooked chickpeas

½ cup sweet onions

½ cup grated carrots

½ cup roasted cashews

Juice of 1 lemon

½ tsp. turmeric

1 tsp. cumin

1 tsp. garlic powder

1 cup rolled oats

Instructions

Combine the olive oil, onions, and carrots into the Air Fryer baking pan and cook them on Air Fry function for 6 minutes at 350 F. Ground the oats and cashews in a food processor. Place in a large bowl. Mix in the chickpeas, lemon juice, and soy sauce.

Add onions and carrots to the bowl with chickpeas. Stir in the remaining ingredients; mix until fully incorporated. Make meatballs out of the mixture. Increase the temperature to 370 F and cook for 12 minutes

SUCCULENT CHICKEN NUGGETS FOR AIR FRYER

Prep time 5 mins Cook Time 10 mins Yields 4 servings

Ingredients

1 lb. chicken tenders

1 tbsp chicken seasoning

1 tbsp olive oil

Instructions

Preheat air fryer to 400°F/200°C. If your air fryer doesn't have this function, let it run empty for 5 minutes.

Add your chicken tenders to a bowl and season with the chicken seasoning. Drizzle the olive oil.

Use a spatula or your hands to coat well the chicken tenders on all sides.

Spray the air fryer basket with non-stick spray and place the chicken pieces in a single layer.

Cook for 10 minutes in the preheated air fryer and flip the tenders halfway.

Transfer to a plate and enjoy with your favorite sides.

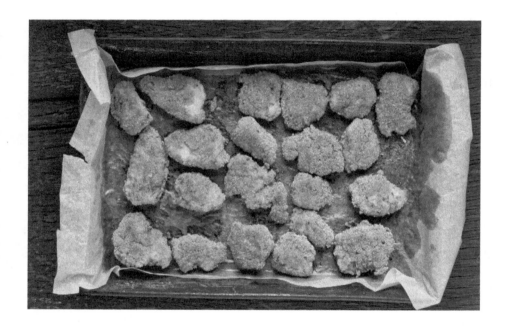

LIGHT CHICKEN AND VEGETABLES WITH AIR FRYER

Prep Time: 5 minutes Cook Time: 15 minutes0 minutes Total Time: 20 minutes Servings: 4 servings

Ingredients

1 pound chicken breast, chopped into bite-size pieces (2-3 medium chicken breasts)

1 cup broccoli florets (fresh or frozen)

1 zucchini chopped

1 cup bell pepper chopped (any colors you like)

1/2 onion chopped

2 clove garlic minced or crushed

2 tablespoons olive oil

1/2 teaspoon EACH garlic powder, chili powder, salt, pepper

1 tablespoon Italian seasoning (or spice blend of choice)

Instructions

Preheat air fryer to 400F.

Chop the veggies and chicken into small bite-size pieces and transfer to a large mixing bowl.

Add the oil and seasoning to the bowl and toss to combine.

Add the chicken and veggies to the preheated air fryer and cook for 10 minutes, shaking halfway, or until the chicken and veggies are charred and chicken is cooked through. If your air fryer is small, you may have to cook them in 2-3 batches.

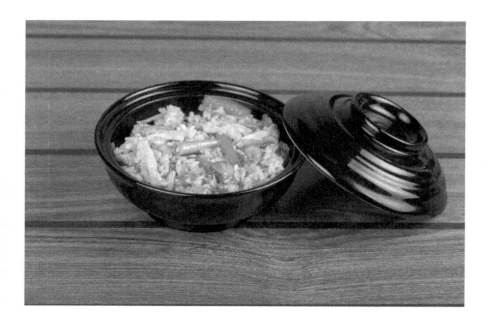

EXQUISITE VEGETABLES BROWNED WITH THE AIR FRYER

prep time: 10 MINUTES

cook time: 20 MINUTES

total time: 30 MINUTES

Ingredients

1 cup broccoli florets

1 cup cauliflower florets

1/2 cup baby carrots

1/2 cup yellow squash, sliced

1/2 cup baby zucchini, sliced

1/2 cup sliced mushrooms

1 small onion, sliced

1/4 cup balsamic vinegar

1 tablespoon olive oil

1 tablespoon minced garlic

1 teaspoon sea salt

1 teaspoon black pepper

1 teaspoon red pepper flakes

1/4 cup parmesan cheese

Instructions

Pre-heat Air Fryer at 400 for 3 minutes.

In a large bowl, put olive oil, balsamic vinegar, garlic, salt and pepper and red pepper flakes.

Super easy and delicious air fryer roasted vegetables that can be made super-fast for dinner in under 20 minutes! #healthyrecipe #vegetables #healthyeats

Whisk together.

Super easy and delicious air fryer roasted vegetables that can be made super-fast for dinner in under 20 minutes! #healthyrecipe #vegetables #healthyeats

Add vegetables and toss to coat.

Super easy and delicious air fryer roasted vegetables that can be made super-fast for dinner in under 20 minutes! #healthyrecipe #vegetables #healthyeats

Add vegetables to Air Fryer basket. Cook for 8 minutes.

Shake vegetables and cook for 6-8 additional minutes.

Super easy and delicious air fryer roasted vegetables that can be made super-fast for dinner in under 20 minutes! #healthyrecipe #vegetables #healthyeats

Add cheese and bake for 1-2 minutes.

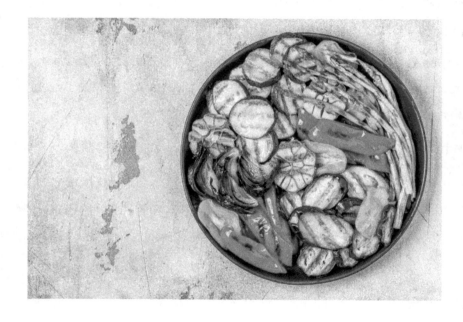

CHICKPEA & CARROT BALLS

Preparation Time: 5 minutes Cooking Time: 20 minutes
Servings: 3

Ingredients

2 tbsp. olive oil

2 tbsp. soy sauce

1 tbsp. flax meal

2 cups cooked chickpeas

½ cup sweet onions

½ cup grated carrots

½ cup roasted cashews

Juice of 1 lemon

½ tsp. turmeric

1 tsp. cumin

1 tsp. garlic powder

1 cup rolled oats

Instructions

Combine the olive oil, onions, and carrots into the Air Fryer baking pan and cook them on Air Fry function for 6 minutes at 350 F. Ground the oats and cashews in a food processor. Place in a large bowl. Mix in the chickpeas, lemon juice, and soy sauce.

Add onions and carrots to the bowl with chickpeas. Stir in the remaining ingredients; mix until fully incorporated. Make meatballs out of the mixture. Increase the temperature to 370 F and cook for 12 minutes.

TASTY AIR FRYER MOZZARELLA STICKS

Prep Time 10 mins

Cook Time 5 mins

Freeze Time 1 hr.

Total Time 1 hr. 15 mins

Servings: 12

Ingredients

12 part-skim cheese sticks

1/4 cup all-purpose flour (gluten-free if needed)

1 large egg

1/3 cup bread crumbs (gluten-free if needed)

1 tsp onion powder

1 tsp garlic powder

1 tsp paprika

1/2 tsp ground black pepper

1/4 tsp salt

nonstick spray

Optional sauces or dips for serving, like marinara

Instructions

To Prepare:

Cut cheese sticks in half to get 24 pieces.

Prepare your breading station: Place flour in the sandwich bag, whisk the egg in a small, shallow dish, then combine bread crumbs and spices in another small, shallow dish.

Place cheese sticks (just a few at a time) in the sandwich bag with the flour. Toss to lightly dust the cheese sticks with flour. Tap off any excessive flour.

Transfer flour-dusted cheese stick to the egg wash and completely coat the cheese stick with egg wash.

Transfer the cheese stick to the bread crumbs and entirely cover. It may be helpful to use a small spoon to help ensure bread crumbs have been poured over every surface.

Place on a silicone mat lined baking dish, then freeze for at least an hour (can be frozen weeks in advance).

To Air Fry:

Preheat air fryer to 385°F. Place frozen mozzarella sticks in a single layer, not touching. Spray the tops with nonstick spray, then cook for 5 minutes.

To Oven Bake:

Preheat oven to 425°F. Place frozen mozzarella sticks on a silicone mat or parchment paper lined baking sheet in a single layer (not touching). Spray the tops with nonstick spray, then cook for 9-10 minutes.

To Serve:

Serve immediately and enjoy while warm. Serve with any of your favorite dipping sauce, like marinara sauce.

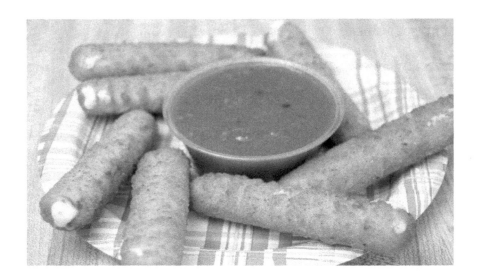

CRISPY AND SOFT JALAPENO POPPERS BALLS

Prep Time   15 minutes

Cook Time   10 minutes a batch

Servings   22 Ball

Ingredients

1 cup Jalapenos diced (about 3)

12 slices bacon

1/2 cup scallions

8 oz cream cheese softened to room temperature

2 cups Sharp Cheddar Cheese shredded

3 tbsp Green Tabasco (green pepper sauce)

Salt and pepper to taste

1/4 tsp garlic powder

1/4 tsp onion powder

2 cups Panko Breadcrumbs

3 eggs

1/2 cup flour

2 tbsp Milk

For Dipping

Sour Cream mixed with Smoky Chipotle Paprika

Marinara

Instructions

Prepare filling ingredients; Cook bacon and chop into small pieces. Dice jalapenos and slice scallions into small pieces.

Mix softened cream cheese, shredded cheddar, jalapenos, scallions, chopped bacon, tabasco, garlic powder, onion powder, salt and pepper (to taste) in a medium bowl.

Line a baking sheet with wax paper. Scoop and roll the mixture into 1.5-2-inch balls, about the size of an ice cream scoop. Place on the baking sheet. (Optional: if your cream cheese mixture is too soft, place your baking sheet and balls in the freezer for 15 minutes to harden a little)

Whisk together your eggs and milk in a small, shallow bowl. Put your flour in a second bowl, and your panko breadcrumbs in a third.

Roll a ball in the flour, dip it in the egg mixture, and then roll it in the breadcrumbs. If you want a thicker crunchy outside, dip the ball in the egg mixture again and roll it in the breadcrumbs a second time. Repeat this process with all of your balls.

Prepare your air fryer with cooking spray and preheat to 400 degrees.

Line your air fryer basket with 4-6 balls, depending on the size of your device, being careful not to cramp them. Fry them for 10-12 minutes, or until golden brown. Repeat in batches of 4-6 until complete.

Serve your air fryer jalapeno popper balls hot, with marinara sauce or sour cream mixed with smoky chipotle paprika for dipping.

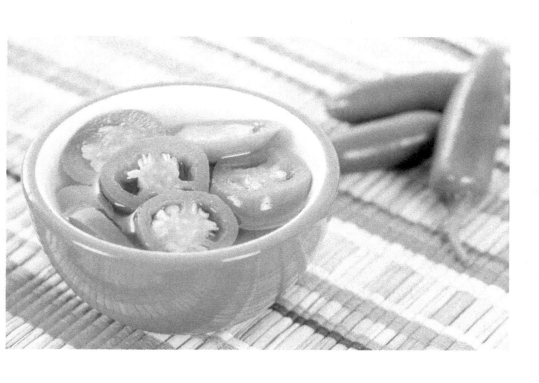

EASY AIR FRYER TUNA STEAKS

YIELD: 2 SERVINGS

PREP TIME

20 minutes

COOK TIME

4 minutes

TOTAL TIME

24 minutes

Ingredients

2 (6 ounce) boneless and skinless yellowfin tuna steaks

1/4 cup soy sauce

2 teaspoons honey

1 teaspoon grated ginger

1 teaspoon sesame oil

1/2 teaspoon rice vinegar

OPTIONAL FOR SERVING

green onions, sliced

sesame seeds

Instructions

Remove the tuna steaks from the fridge.

In a large bowl, combine the soy sauce, honey, grated ginger, sesame oil, and rice vinegar.

Place tuna steaks in the marinade and let marinate for 20-30 minutes covered in the fridge.

Preheat air fryer to 380 degrees and then cook the tuna steaks in one layer for 4 minutes.

Let the air fryer tuna steaks rest for a minute or two, then slice, and enjoy immediately! Garnish with green onions and/or sesame seeds if desired

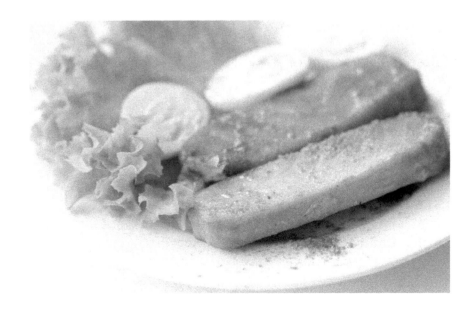

AIR FRYER LEMON SHRIMP

YIELD: 4 SERVINGS

PREP TIME

5 minutes

COOK TIME

8 minutes

TOTAL TIME

13 minutes

Ingredients

1-pound medium raw shrimp, peeled and deveined

1/2 cup olive oil

2 tablespoons lemon juice

1 teaspoon black pepper

1/2 teaspoon salt

Instructions

Preheat your air fryer to 400 degrees.

Place the shrimp in a Ziploc bag with the olive oil, lemon juice, salt, and pepper. Carefully combine all ingredients.

Add parchment paper round (if using) and place the raw shrimp inside the air fryer in one layer.

Cook for about 8 minutes, shaking the basket halfway through. The shrimp are done when the shells turn pink and the shrimp is just slightly white, but still a little opaque.

Remove the lemon pepper shrimp from the air fryer, serve with pasta if desired, and enjoy

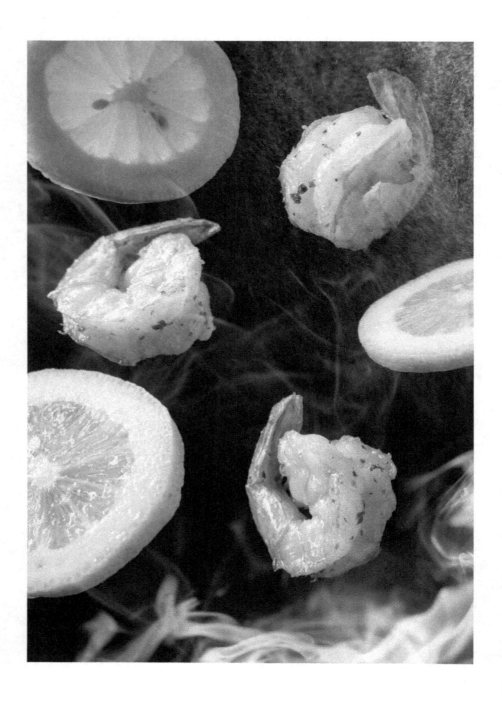

DELICIOUS AIR FRYER BACON-WRAPPED STUFFED JALAPENOS

YIELD: 6 SERVINGS

PREP TIME

10 minutes

COOK TIME

14 minutes

TOTAL TIME

24 minutes

Ingredients

12 Jalapenos

8 ounces of cream cheese, room temperature or slightly soft

1/2 cup shredded cheddar cheese

1/4 teaspoon garlic powder

1/8 teaspoon onion powder

12 slices of bacon, thinly cut

87

salt and pepper to taste

Instructions

Cut the jalapenos in half, remove the stems, and remove the seeds and membranes. The more membrane you leave, the spicier the jalapenos will be.

Add cream cheese, shredded cheddar cheese, garlic powder, onion powder, salt, and pepper in a bowl. Mix to combine.

Using a small spoon, scoop the cream mixture into each jalapeno filling it just to the top.

Preheat air fryer to 350 degrees for about 3 minutes.

Cut each slice of bacon in half.

Wrap each jalapeno half in one piece of bacon.

Place the bacon-wrapped stuffed jalapenos in the air fryer in an even layer making sure they do not touch.

Air fry at 350 degrees for 14-16 minutes, until bacon is thoroughly cooked.

Enjoy immediately or refrigerate for up to 3 days, reheating before eating.

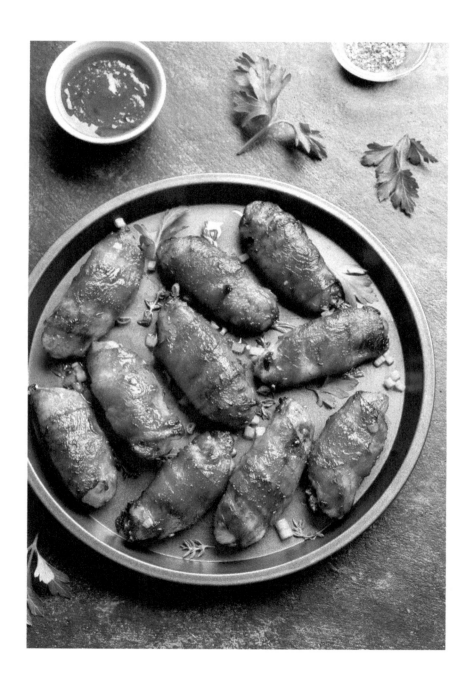

KETO AIR FRYER GARLIC CHICKEN BREAST

YIELD: 4 SERVINGS

PREP TIME

2 minutes

COOK TIME

10 minutes

TOTAL TIME

12 minutes

Ingredients

4 boneless chicken breasts

2 tablespoons butter

1/4 teaspoon garlic powder

1/2 teaspoon salt

1/4 teaspoon pepper

Instructions

Place boneless chicken breasts on a cutting board.

Melt butter in the microwave and add in garlic powder, salt, and pepper. Mix to combine.

Coat chicken with butter mixture on both sides.

Place chicken in the air fryer in one single layer.

Cook chicken at 380 degrees for 10-15 minutes, flipping halfway. The chicken is done once the chicken reads 165 degrees at its thickest part.

Let chicken rest for 5 minutes.

Enjoy immediately or refrigerate and enjoy cold or using reheated directions above.

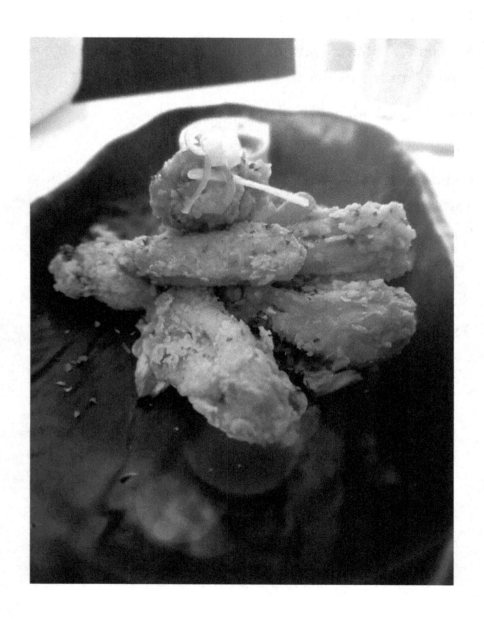

RIBEYE STEAK FRIES

YIELD: 2 SERVINGS

PREP TIME

5 minutes

COOK TIME

10 minutes

ADDITIONAL TIME

30 minutes

TOTAL TIME

45 minutes

Ingredients

8-ounce ribeye steak, about 1-inch thick

1 tablespoon McCormick Montreal Steak Seasoning

Instructions

Remove the ribeye steak from the fridge and season with the Montreal Steak seasoning. Let steak rest for about 20 minutes to come to room temperature (to get a more tender juicy steak).

Preheat your air fryer to 400 degrees.

Place the ribeye steak in the air fryer and cook for 10-12 minutes, until it reaches 130-135 degrees for medium rare. Cook for an additional 5 minutes for medium-well.

Remove the steak from the air fryer and let rest at least 5 minutes before cutting to keep the juices inside the steak then enjoy!

How to preheat steak in the air fryer:

1. Preheat your air fryer to 350 degrees.

2. Cook steak in the air fryer for 3 to 5 minutes until heated thoroughly, let sit fot 5 minutes, then enjoy!

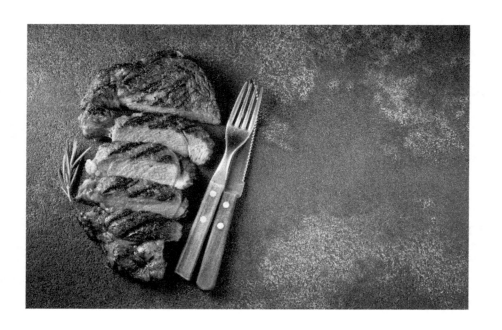

AIR FRYER LEMON COD LOINS

YIELD: 4 SERVINGS

PREP TIME

10 minutes

COOK TIME

10 minutes

TOTAL TIME

20 minutes

Ingredients

4 cod loins

4 tablespoons butter, melted

6 cloves of garlic, minced

2 tablespoons lemon juice (1 lemon)

1 teaspoon dried dill (or 2 tablespoons fresh dill, chopped)

1/2 teaspoon salt

Instructions

Preheat your air fryer to 370 degrees.

Mix the butter, garlic, lemon juice, dill, and salt in a bowl.

Add a cod loin into the bowl coating it completely. Lightly press the garlic into the cod so it doesn't fall off when cooking. Repeat with remaining cod pieces.

Place all the cod loins into the air fryer in one layer not touching.

Cook for 10 minutes then carefully remove from the air fryer.

Garnish the cod with more lemon juice or butter if desired and enjoy!

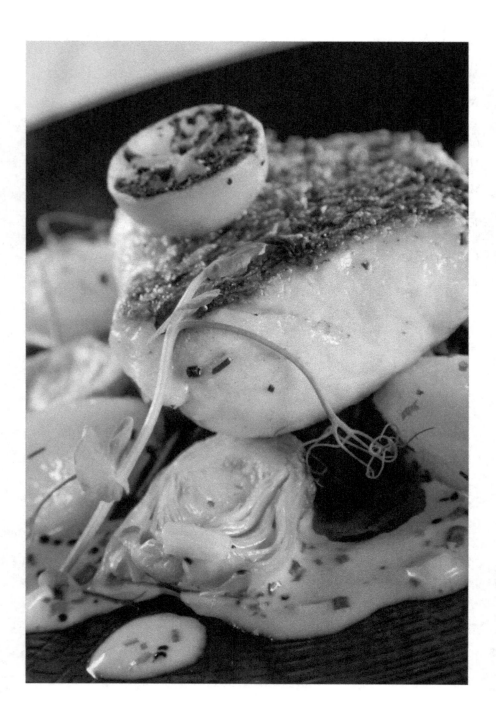

AIR FRYER CHICKEN FAJITAS

Yield: 4 servings

Prep time 10 minutes

Cook time 10 minutes

Total time 20 minutes

Ingredients

1/2 pound boneless and skinless chicken breasts, cut into 1/2-inch-wide strips

1 large red or yellow bell pepper, cut into strips

1 medium red onion, cut into strips

1 tablespoon Mazola Corn Oil

1 tablespoon chili powder

2 teaspoons lime juice

1 teaspoon cumi

Salt and pepper to taste

OPTIONAL

pinch of cayenne pepper

tortillas for serving

Instructions

Preheat your air fryer to 370 degrees.

Put the chicken strips, bell pepper, onion, Mazola Corn Oil, chili powder, lime juice, cumin, salt and pepper, and cayenne pepper (if using) in a bowl and mix.

Place the chicken fajitas in the air fryer and cook for 10-13 minutes, shaking the basket halfway through. The fajitas are done when the chicken hits 165 degrees F at its thickest point.

Remove the fajitas from the air fryer, warm tortillas if needed, and enjoy!

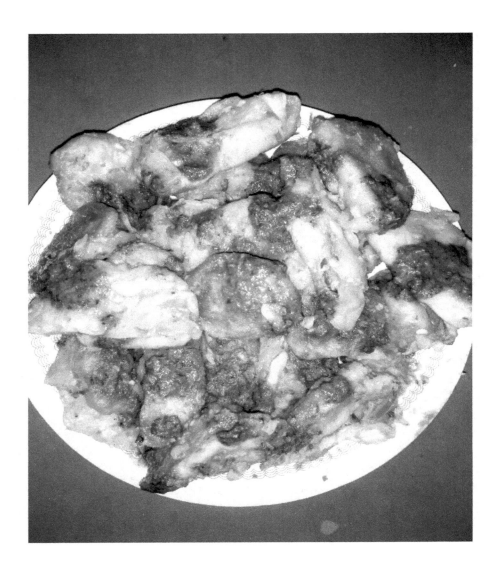

SAUSAGE BREAKFAST PATTIES

YIELD: 4 SERVINGS

COOK TIME

6 minutes

TOTAL TIME

6 minutes

Ingredients

8 raw sausage breakfast Pattie

Instructions

Preheat your air fryer to 370 degrees.

Place the raw sausage patties in the air fryer in one layer not touching.

Cook for 6-8 minutes, until they reach 160 degrees. *

Remove from the air fryer and enjoy!

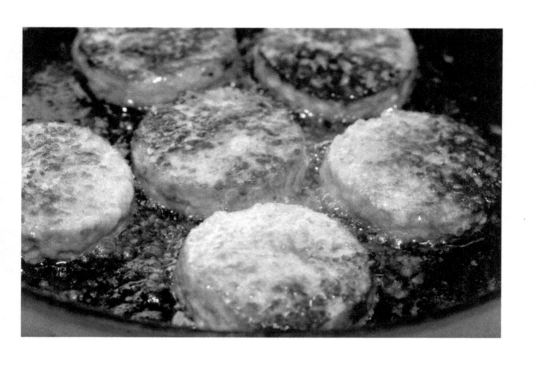

AIR FRYER SALMON FILLETS

YIELD: 2 SERVINGS

PREP TIME

5 minutes

COOK TIME

10 minutes

TOTAL TIME

15 minutes

Ingredients

2 (6-ounce) boneless, skin-on salmon fillets (preferably wild-caught)

2 tablespoons butter, melted

1 teaspoon garlic, minced

1 teaspoon fresh Italian parsley, chopped (or 1/4 teaspoon dried)

salt and pepper to taste

Instructions

Preheat the air fryer to 360 degrees.

Season the fresh salmon with salt and pepper then mix together the melted butter, garlic, and parsley in a bowl.

Baste the salmon fillets with the garlic butter mixture and carefully place the salmon inside the air fryer side-by-side with the skin side down.

Cook for approximately 10 minutes until salmon flakes easily with a knife or fork.

Eat immediately or store up to 3 days using the reheating directions below.

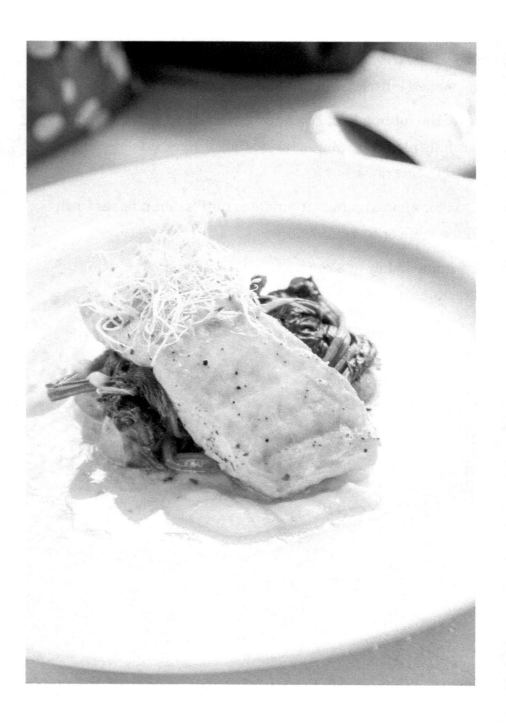

AIR FRIED CHICKEN DRUMSTICKS BBQ SAUCE

YIELD: 5 SERVINGS

PREP TIME

5 minutes

COOK TIME

25 minutes

TOTAL TIME

30 minutes

Ingredients

5-6 chicken drumsticks

1/8 cup extra virgin olive oil

1/2 teaspoon garlic powder

1/4 teaspoon paprika

1/4 teaspoon onion powder

1/4 teaspoon salt

1/8 teaspoon pepper

1/2 cup BBQ sauce (I prefer Sweet Baby Ray's)

Instructions

Preheat your air fryer to 400 degrees.

Pat dry chicken drumsticks.

Mix together the olive oil, garlic powder, paprika, onion powder, salt and pepper, and cayenne pepper (if using).

Coat the chicken drumsticks with oil mixture and massage into the drumsticks for a few minutes to help keep the flavor in.

Add chicken drumsticks to the air fryer in one single layer and cook for 15 minutes.

Flip chicken and cook for another 5 minutes.

Baste chicken with BBQ sauce, flip, then baste other side of chicken with BBQ sauce.

Cook until chicken has an internal temperature of 165 degrees, about 3-5 more minutes.

Remove from the air fryer, baste additional BBQ sauce if desired and enjoy!

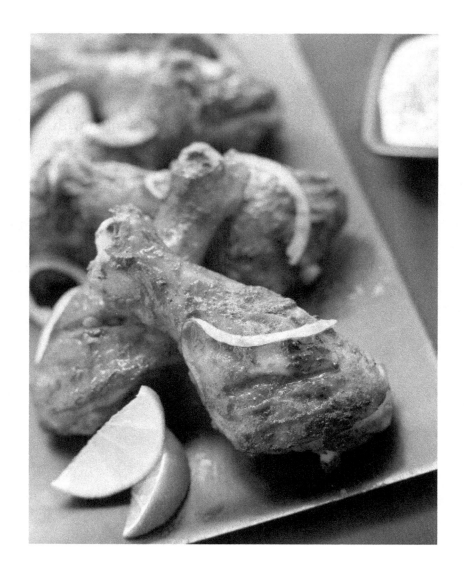

Conclusion

Nowadays, having an air fryer in the house is an added value.

It is a practical and very flexible kitchen appliance with which you can do a lot. New cooking ideas can be experimented with while keeping calories and fat intake under control.

Of course, a hot air fryer is not a diet device that will make you lose weight, but it will certainly not make you give up good frying for good.

Many people take advantage of this new form of preparation., to cook meat fish vegetables or others.

Now you can fry all this without being afraid of enlarging the liver.

If you're into low-fat eating, you should definitely take a look at hot air fryers. The benefits will be great.

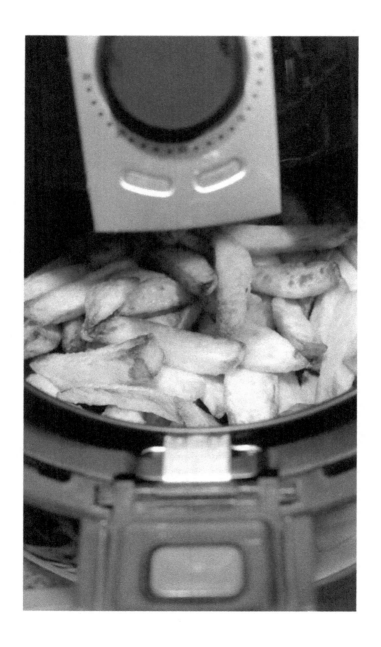

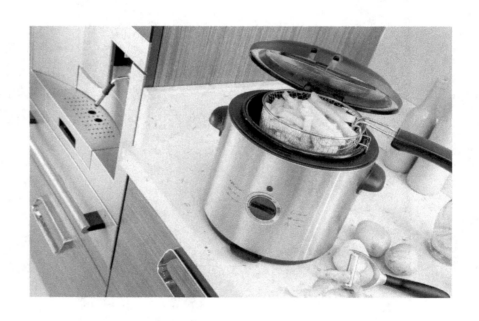

AIR FRYER HEALTHY COOKBOOK

Truly Healthy Fried Recipes with Low Salt and Low Fat, Ideal Cooking to Prevent Disease, Control Weight and Live Well While Eating. Keeps You and Your Family Healthy, Satisfies Splurges Without Any Guilt.

Violet H.Scott

Introduction

Tired of depriving yourself of tasty fried foods because the pounds are adding up and your liver is screaming for help? The solution exists, and it is to use an air fryer- This is a fantastic and innovative appliance that makes it easy and fast to cook delicious and healthy meals,

that makes it easy and quick to cook delicious and healthy meals.

Easy to clean and store, convenience is one of its strengths.

Goodbye oil splatters, on the walls, on the floor. Not to mention the time it takes to deglaze the used product after cooking.

In a short period of time, the air fryer

will prepare your meal, whether it's chicken, steak, fish or vegetables,

frying them perfectly.

In addition to savory dishes, you can also use an air fryer with excellent results for cakes, tarts and even bread.

Its great advantage is the fact that it keeps the nutritional content intact compared to cooking with a classic fryer. High cooking temperatures deprive food of much of what our bodies need.

The difference is that when food is prepared in an air fryer, it is only cooked to the safe temperatures appropriate for your health and food. It prepares healthy meals with less time, more control and healthier results. It is the most efficient way to cook.

Hot air replaces oil, creating a crisp, delicious crust.

It will cook evenly, thanks to the perfect heat distribution aided by the fan.

The calories of typical fried foods will be a distant memory, with the absence or minimal amount of added oil, they will be reduced dramatically, without going to the expense of crispiness.

Your food will taste just like fried food, without the oil.

Equipped with a thermostat that comes with protection against overheating, there will be no danger of burning your food. There's also a food weight indicator, so you'll know the exact amount you're preparing, and a timer with an automatic shut-off feature, so you can safely do other activities while cooking.

Cooking takes place evenly, thanks to the perfect distribution of heat aided by the fan.

The calories of typical fried foods will be a distant memory, with the absence or minimal amount of oil added, will be reduced dramatically, without going to the expense of crispness.

Your food will taste just like fried food, without the oil.

Air fryer recipes

PARIKA POTATO FRIES
PAPRIKA POTATO FRIES

To prepare

5 minutes

Prepare

20 minutes

Number of persons 4

Ingredients

750 gr sweet potato, about 4 pieces

1 tbsp chili powder

1 tbsp paprika powder

1 tbsp fine salt

Instructions

1. Heat the Airfryer to 180 ° C.

2. Peel the sweet potatoes and cut into equal slices of about 1 cm. Cut 1 cm wide fries from these slices.

3. Mix with chili powder, paprika and salt and bake in the Airfryer for 15 to 20 minutes.

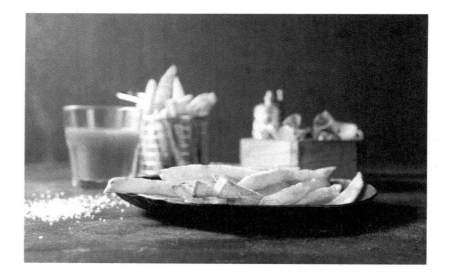

OVEN ZUCCHINI WITH SMOKED SALMON

Preparation time 15 minutes

Preparation time 45 minutes

Total time 1 hour

Ingredients

1 zucchini, at least 300 grams

200 grams of smoked salmon

3 tablespoons of mild olive oil

1 teaspoon of black pepper from the pepper mill

1/2 teaspoon of Celtic sea salt

1 large clove of garlic, finely chopped

80 grams créme fraiche

3 eggs, size large

75 grams of grated grana padano

☐handful of finely chopped fresh coriander

Instructions

Set your oven to 180 degrees to preheat. If you use an Airfryer, it also goes at 180 degrees.

Cut the zucchini into small cubes and the smoked salmon into strips.

In a frying pan, fry the garlic lightly brown in the mild olive oil and then add the zucchini cubes. Stir fry until the zucchini is almost cooked.

Turn off the heat and add the smoked salmon and coriander to the zucchini.

Meanwhile, in a bowl, stir together the eggs, creme fraiche and 50 grams of grana padano to a smooth batter.

Crumble your baking paper and place it in your baking tin.

Spoon the zucchini and smoked salmon mix into the baking tin. Pour the batter over it. Sprinkle the remaining 25 grams of Grana Padano over the quiche.

Bake in the center of the oven for 20-25 minutes.

If you use an Airfryer, the baking time is around 15 minutes at 180 degrees

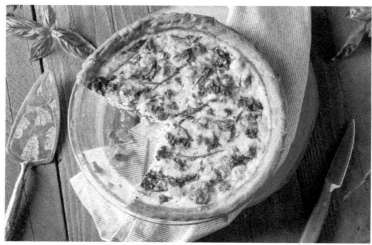

AIR FRYER HALLOUMI

Prep time 3 mins

Cook time 10 mins

Ingredients

1 lb halloumi (450 g)

½ cup breadcrumbs (8 tablespoons)

1 egg

½ teaspoon salt

½ teaspoon garlic powder

Instructions

Slice the halloumi into thick fries.

Crack the egg into a bowl, and whisk until it's combined. In another bowl, add the breadcrumbs, salt and garlic powder.

Use a fork to dip each halloumi stick individually into the whisked egg, then into the breadcrumbs. The cheese should be coated with the breading on all sides. Repeat with each fry.

Preheat your air fryer to 180 °C/ 355 °F. Then, add the breaded halloumi sticks to the air fryer basket. Make sure to leave room between each stick to allow the halloumi to cook evenly.

Air fry the halloumi fries for 8-10 minutes, turning them once halfway through the cooking time. Serve them immediately while they are still hot.

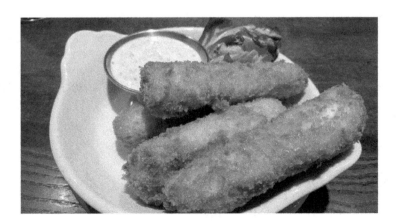

LOW CARB SALMON CAKES

PREP:35 minutes

COOK:15 minutes

TOTAL:50 minutes

Ingredients

1 lb ALDI Fresh Atlantic Salmon Side (half a side)

1/4 Cup Avocado, mashed

1/4 Cup Cilantro, diced + additional for garnish

1 1/2 tsp Yellow curry powder

1/2 tsp l Sea Salt Grinder

1/4 Cup + 4 tsp Tapioca Starch, divided (40g) *Read notes for lower carb version

2 Simply Nature Organic Cage Free Brown Eggs

1/2 Cup Coconut Flakes (30g)

Coconut Oil, melted (for brushing)

For the Greens:

2 tsp Coconut Oil, melted

6 Cups Arugula & Spinach Mix, tightly packed

Pinch of Sea Salt Grinder

Instructions

Remove the skin from the salmon, dice the flesh, and add it into a large bowl.

Add in the avocado, cilantro, curry powder, sea salt and stir until well mixed. Then, stir in 4 tsp of the tapioca starch until well incorporated.

Line a baking sheet with parchment paper. Form the salmon into 8, 1/4 cup-sized patties, just over 1/2 inch thick, and place them onto the pan. Freeze for 20 minutes so they are easier to work with.

While the patties freeze, pre-heat your Air Fryer to 400 degrees for 10 minutes, rubbing the basket with coconut oil. Additionally, whisk the eggs and place them into a shallow plate. Place the remaining 1/4 cup of Tapioca starch and the coconut flakes in separate shallow plates as well.

Once the patties have chilled, dip one into the tapioca starch, making sure it's fully covered. Then, dip it into the egg, covering it entirely, and gently brushing off any excess. Finally, press just the top and sides of the cake into the coconut flakes and place it, coconut flake-side up, into the air fryer. Repeat with all cakes. **

Gently brush the tops with a little bit of melted coconut oil (optional, but recommended) and cook until the outside is golden brown and crispy, and the inside is juicy and tender, about 15 minutes. Note: the patties will stick to the Air Fryer basked a little, so use a sharp-edged spatula to remove them.

When the cakes have about 5 minutes left to cook, heat the coconut oil up in a large pan on medium heat. Add in the Arugula and Spinach Mix, and a pinch of salt, and cook, stirring constantly, until the greens JUST begin to wilt, only 30 seconds - 1 minute.

Divide the greens between 4 plates, followed by the salmon cakes. Garnish with extra cilantro and DEVOUR!

If You Want to Bake In The Oven:

Preheat your oven to 400 degrees and line a baking sheet with parchment paper, placing a cooling rack on top of the pan. Rub the cooling rack with coconut oil.

Place the patties, coconut-side up, onto the cooling rack and bake for 15-17 minutes until crispy. NOTE: we liked these better in the air fryer, as they do get a little crispier, but they are still good in the oven!

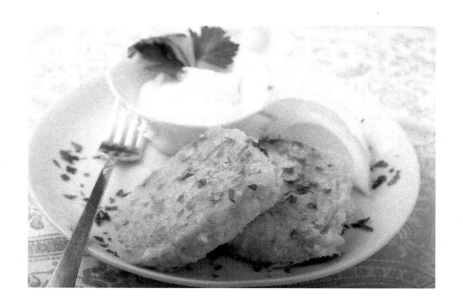

DELICIOUS POTATO CAULIFLOWER PATTIES

Prep Time: 15

Cook Time: 20

Total Time: 35 minutes

Yield: 7

Ingredients

1 medium to large sweet potato, peeled

2 cup cauliflower florets

1 green onion, chopped.

1 tsp minced garlic

2 tbsp organic ranch seasoning mix or dairy seasoning mix of choice

1 cup packed cilantro (fresh)

1/2 tsp chili powder

1/4 tsp cumin

2 tbsp arrowroot starch or gluten free flour of choice

1/4 cup ground flaxseed

1/4 cup sunflower seeds (or pumpkin seeds)

1/4 tsp Kosher Salt and pepper (or to taste)

Dipping sauce of choice

Instructions

Pre-heat oven to 400F. Line a baking sheet (or oil) and set aside.

Next cut your peeled sweet potato into smaller pieces. Place in a food processor or blender and pulse until the larger pieces are broken up.

Add in your cauliflower, onion, and garlic and pulse again.

Add in the sunflower seeds, flaxseed, arrowroot (or flour), cilantro, and remaining seasonings. Pulse or place on medium until a thick batter is formed. See blog for picture.

Place batter in larger bowl. Scoop 1/4 cup of the batter out at a time and form into patties about 1.5 inches thick. Place on baking sheet.

Repeat until you have about 7-10 patties.

Chill in freeze for 10 minutes so the patties can set.

Once set, place patties in oven for 20 minutes, flipping halfway. If you made your patties extra thick, they could take closer to 25 minutes.

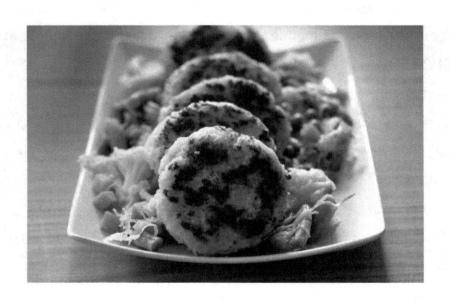

AIR FRYER ITALIAN ZUCCHINI CHIPS

Prep Time15 minutes

Cook Time10 minutes

Total Time25 minutes

Servings5

Ingredients

1 large zucchini Mine weighed 1.5 pounds.

1/2 cup all-purpose flour

1 teaspoon Italian Seasoning

1 teaspoon Smoked Paprika or your favorite seasoning

1/4 cup finely shredded parmesan cheese

salt and pepper to taste

2 eggs, beaten

1 1/2-2 cups breadcrumb I used panko breadcrumbs.

cooking oil spray

Instructions

Spray the air fryer basket with cooking oil.

Add eggs, flour, and breadcrumbs to separate bowls.

Slice the zucchini into chips about 1/4 of an inch thick. You can also use a mandolin for precise slicing. You want to get the zucchini chips all about the same size so that they cook at an even temperature.

Season the flour with salt and pepper to taste, and paprika and add shredded parmesan.

Dip the zucchini in the flour, then egg, and then the breadcrumbs and place in the air fryer. Make sure to coat the chip fully in the eggs so that the breadcrumbs will stick.

Keep a moist towel nearby because your hands will get sticky.

Spray the zucchini chips with cooking oil spray using a spray bottle.

Air Fry for 5 minutes on 400 degrees.

Open and flip the chips. Spray with additional oil and cook for an additional 4-7 minutes on 400 degrees. The zucchini chips will brown by 8 minutes, if you like them crispy, cook them a little longer. Mine were ready around 10-11 minutes.

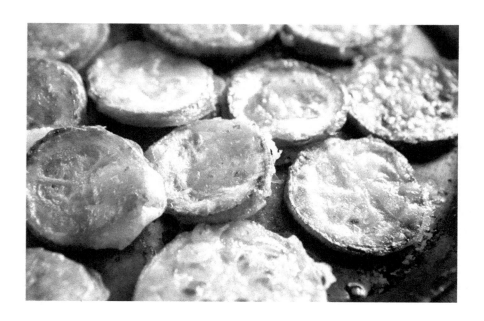

AIR FRYER JUMBO SHRIMP

Ingredients

2 pounds jumbo cooked shrimp, peeled and deveined

4 cloves garlic, minced

2/3 cup parmesan cheese, grated

1 teaspoon pepper

1/2 teaspoon oregano

1 teaspoon basil

1 teaspoon onion powder

2 tablespoons olive oil

Lemon, quartered

Instructions

In a large bowl, combine garlic, parmesan cheese, pepper, oregano, basil, onion powder and olive oil.

Gently toss shrimp in mixture until evenly-coated.

Spray air fryer basket with non-stick spray and place shrimp in basket.

Cook at 350 degrees for 8-10 minutes or until seasoning on shrimp is browned.

Squeeze the lemon over the shrimp before serving.

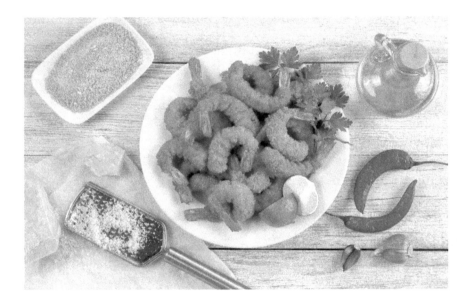

LOW CARB RANCH STEAK NUGGETS

Ingredients

1 pound venison steak or beef steak, cut into chunks.

1 large Egg(s), Organic Pasture Raised

Lard or palm oil for frying

Keto Breading

1/2 cup grated parmesan cheese

1/2 cup pork panko

1/2 teaspoon Homemade Seasoned Salt

Chipotle Ranch Dip

1/4 cup mayonnaise

1/4 cup Sour Cream (organic, cultured)

1+ teaspoon chipotle pastes to taste

1/2 teaspoon Homemade Ranch Dressing & Dip Mix

1/4 medium lime, juiced

Instructions

For the Chipotle Ranch Dip: Combine all ingredients, mix well. 1 teaspoon of chipotle paste yields a medium-spice version, use more or less according to your own taste preferences. I encourage you to use my homemade ranch dressing and dip mix, it's superior to any store brought version. Refrigerate at least 30 minutes before serving, will keep for up to 1 week.

Combine Pork Panko, parmesan cheese and seasoned salt - again use my homemade not the store-bought stuff. Set aside.

Beat 1 egg. place beaten egg 1 bowl and breading mix in another.

Dip chunks of steak in egg, then breading. Place on a wax paper lined sheet pan or plate.

FREEZE breaded raw steak bites for 30 minutes before frying. This helps to ensure that the breading will NOT LIFT when fried.

Heat Lard to roughly 325 degrees F. Working in batches as necessary, fry steak nuggets (from frozen or chilled) until browned, about 2-3 minutes.

Transfer to a paper towel lined plate, season with a sprinkle of salt and serve with Chipotle Ranch.

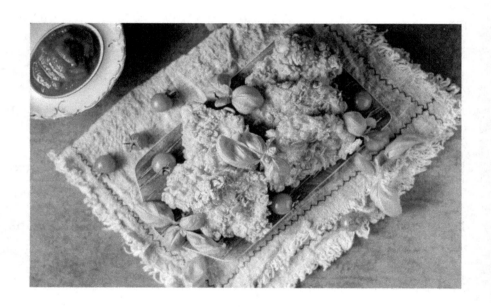

AIR FRYER SALMON FILLETS TERIYAKI

prep time: 5 MINS cook time: 8 MINS marinade: 15 MINS total time: 28 MINS servings: 3

Ingredients

1/3+1/4 cup Keto Teriyaki Sauce, see notes

16.5 oz. salmon fillets (3 slices at 5.5 oz per fillet), 1.5-inch at thickest

1/8 tsp xanthan gum

Toasted white sesame seeds, sprinkle optional

1 bulb scallion, chopped

Instructions

For the teriyaki sauce:

Follow this keto teriyaki sauce recipe instructions to prepare the sauce but do not add the xanthan gum thickener. Let the sauce cool to room temperature.

Teriyaki salmon marinade:

In a small baking tray or casserole dish that's just big enough to fill in all the salmon pieces, pour over ⅓ cup of the teriyaki sauce and marinate the fish skin side up for 15-20 minutes.

Air fried the salmon:

Line the air fryer basket with a thin layer of parchment paper or an air fryer liner. Slightly drip off the marinade and place the fish, side skin down, in the basket and with some gap between the fillets. Discard the marinade.

Air fry at 400F for 7 to 9 minutes. The exact time will depend on the thickness of the fish and your appliance. Mine was done at 7 minutes for medium-rare and 8 minutes for medium.

To thicken the teriyaki sauce, take ¼ cup of the sauce and add it to a small sauce pot. Bring it to a low simmer. Gradually and slowly sprinkle in 1/8 tsp xanthan gum while whisking at the same time to prevent clumps.

Teriyaki homemade sauce in a white and blue cup

The fish will be nearly opaque when cut into, at 120F (49C) at the thickest part. You can peek into the thickest part with a sharp knife or fork. It should flake easily, but still has a little translucency in the center.

Transfer the fishes to a plater. Glaze the salmon with teriyaki sauce. Sprinkle with toasted sesame seeds, if using, and scallions. Remove the skin before serving. I recommend serving them warm.

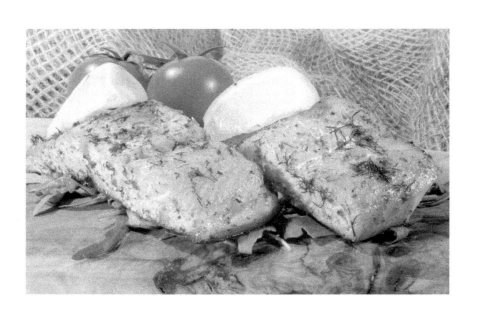

AIR FRYER AVOCADO

Servings: 35 fries

Calories: 46 kcal

Ingredients

2 large avocados

½ cup unsweetened almond milk, may also sub with 1 large egg if not vegan

½ cup superfine blanched almond flour

For the coating:

1 cup unsweetened toasted shredded coconut, OR sub with crushed Simple Mills Grain-Free Sea Salt Almond Flour Crackers (or other favorite grain-free crackers like Hu's Kitchen Grain-Free Crackers)

1.5 tbsp Cajun seasoning spice mix OR smoked paprika

Salt and pepper

For the optional dip:

⅓ cup vegan mayo

1 tbsp lemon juice

½ tbsp Cajun seasoning

Salt and pepper to taste

Instructions

Use a large knife to cut your avocados in half and remove the pit from the middle. Cut the avocado into wedges or "fries".

Homemade Guacamole - this quick and simple recipe is the perfect easy party dip with tortilla chips or along with tacos or by the spoonful. Best of all, only 6 ingredients to make for your next Mexican-inspired meal.

Oven Method

Preheat oven to 400F. Line a large baking sheet with parchment paper.

Gather three wide shallow bowls. Place the almond milk in one bowl, the almond flour in the next bowl and combine the coating ingredients in the the third bowl.

Take one avocado slice, place it in the flour. Make sure it is fully coated in flour then gently shake to get rid of any excess flour.

Place it in the almond milk and again make sure it is fully coated and wet. You will find it easier if you use one hand for the first two steps and then the other hand for the breading, so you don't get too messy!

Finally place it in the coconut breading, making sure it is fully coated, then place on the baking pan.

Repeat until all the slices are coated. Place the baking sheet in the oven for 15-20 minutes until turning golden brown.

FOR THE DIP:

Make the dip by mixing all the ingredients together. Enjoy with the avocado fries!

Air Fryer Method

Place the breaded avocado sticks in a single layer in the air fryer basket, you will have to work in batches.

Lightly coat with cooking spray and cook for 8-12 minutes at 375F, or until golden and crispy, flipping halfway through.

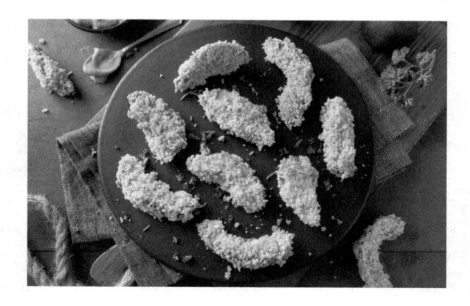

Creamy Chicken, Rice, And Peas

Preparation Time: 10 minutes Cooking Time: 30 minutes
Servings: 4

Ingredients

1 lb. chicken breasts	½ cup white wine
1 cup white rice	¼ cup heavy cream
Salt and black pepper	1 cup chicken stock
1 tbsp. olive oil	¼ cup parsley
Three garlic cloves	2 cups peas
One yellow onion	One and ½ cups parmesan

Directions:

Spice chicken breasts with pepper and salt, sprinkle half oil over them. Rub well and place in the air fryer, then cook at 360 °F for 6 minutes.

Heat pan with remaining oil over high heat. Add garlic, wine, onion, stock, pepper, and heavy cream, salt, stir, simmer, and cook for 9 minutes.

Put chicken breasts in a heatproof dish and add peas, cream mix, rice, and toss. Sprinkle parsley and parmesan all over, put in the air fryer, and cook at 420 °F for 10 minutes.

Divide between plates and serve hot while.

AIR FRYER KETO QUESO FUNDIDO

Prep Time: 10 minutes Cook Time: 25 minutes Stand Time: 30 minutes Total Time: 35 minutes

Ingredients

4 ounces (113.4 g) Mexican-style chorizo, casings removed

1 cup (160 g) onions, chopped

1 tablespoon (1 tablespoon) Minced Garlic

1 cup (149 g) diced tomatoes

2 (2) jalepenos, diced

2 teaspoons (2 teaspoons) Ground Cumin

2 cups (473.18 g) grated Oaxaca cheese or Mozzarella

1/2 cup (121 g) Half and Half

Instructions

In a 6 x 3 heatproof pan, mix together the chorizo, onion, garlic, tomatoes, jalepenos and ground cumin. Place pan in the air fryer basket.

Set the air fryer to 400F for 15 minutes or until the sausage is cooked. Halfway through cooking, stir the mixture to break up the sausage.

Add the cheese and half and half and stir again.

Set air fryer to 320F for 10 minutes until the cheese has melted.

Serve with tortillas or chips.

To further reduce carbs, cut onions in half, and use cherry tomatoes instead of regular tomatoes

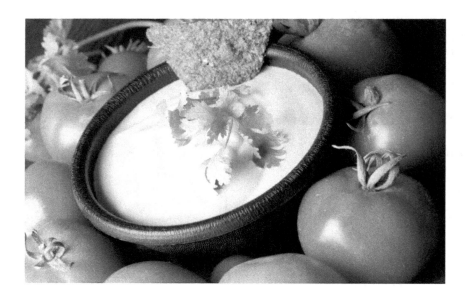

AIR FRYER TILAPIA FILLETS

Prep Time: 10

Cook Time: 8

Total Time: 18

Yield: 4 servings

Ingredients

1 teaspoon lemon juice

1 teaspoon dried oregano

1 teaspoon garlic powder

1 teaspoon salt

4 (6 ounces) tilapia fillets

olive oil spray

Instructions

Start by making the rub, mix together the lemon juice, oregano, garlic powder, and salt.

Then rub the spices onto the fish. (Both sides)

Spray the fish with olive oil spray, and then place into the air fryer basket or oven. Set the temperature for 400 degrees F, for 4 minutes, after 4 minutes, flip (spray again) and add another 4 minutes.

Plate, serve, and enjoy!

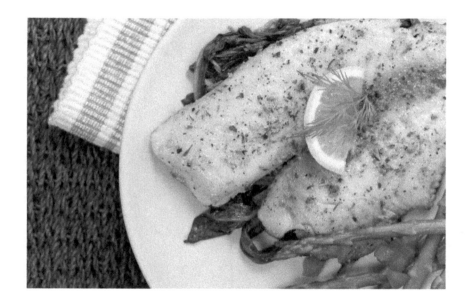

AIR FRYER FLANK STEAK WITH CHIMICHURRI SAUCE

Prep Time: 10

Cook Time: 10

Total Time: 20

Yield: 4 servings

Ingredients

2 pounds flank steak

Chimichurri Sauce:

1/2 cup diced parsley

1/2 cup diced cilantro

1/2 onion

1 teaspoon salt

1/2 teaspoon black pepper

1 teaspoon garlic

1/2 teaspoon red pepper flakes

1/3 cup olive oil

2 tablespoons red wine vinegar

Instructions

The first thing I do when making steak, let the meat rest at room temperature for AT LEAST 30 minutes.

Start by preheating the air fryer, steak is one of the few recipes, that I preheat the air fryer for. But the meat will come out better, so turn the air fryer oven'/basket on for 5 minutes at 400 degrees F.

Then rub the olive oil or butter all over the steak, and season with salt and pepper.

Set the steaks in the air fryer for 6 minutes, then flip and air fry for another 6 minutes.

Again, per Bobby Flay, let the steak rest for at least 5 minutes.

Plate, serve, and enjoy!

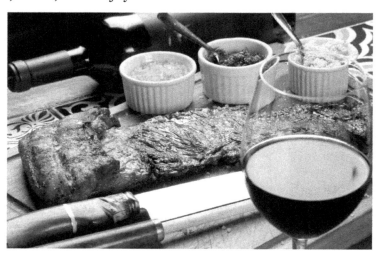

AIR FRYER SCALLOPS WITH TOMATO CREAM SAUCE

Prep Time: 5 minutes Cook Time: 10 minutes Total Time: 15 minutes

Servings: 2

Ingredients

3/4 cup (178.5 g) Heavy Whipping Cream

1 tablespoon (1 tablespoon) Tomato Paste

1 tablespoon (1 tablespoon) chopped fresh basil

1 teaspoon (1 teaspoon) Minced Garlic

1/2 teaspoon (0.5 teaspoon) Kosher Salt

1/2 teaspoon (0.5 teaspoon) Ground Black Pepper

1 12 oz (1 12 oz) Frozen Spinach, thawed and drained

8 (8) jumbo sea scallops

Cooking Oil Spray

additional salt and pepper to season scallops

Instructions

Spray a 7-inch heatproof pan, and place the spinach in an even layer at the bottom.

Spray both sides of the scallops with vegetable oil, sprinkle a little more salt and pepper on them, and place scallops in the pan on top of the spinach.

In a small bowl, mix together the cream, tomato paste, basil, garlic, salt and pepper and pour over the spinach and scallops.

Set the air fryer to 350F for 10 minutes until the scallops are cooked through to an internal temperature of 135F and the sauce is hot and bubbling. Serve immediately.

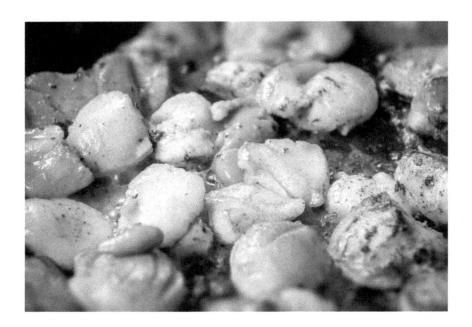

CRISPY AIR FRYER BRUSSELS SPROUTS

Prep Time

5 mins

Cook Time

15 mins

Total Time

20 mins

Servings: 4 servings Calories: 155kcal

Ingredients

2 cups Brussel sprouts

2 Tablespoons coconut oil

1/4 cup parmesan cheese grated

1/4 cup almonds sliced and crushed

2 Tablespoons everything bagel seasoning

Sea salt to taste

Instructions

Add Brussel sprouts to a medium saucepan with 2 cups of water, cover and cook over medium heat for 8-10 minutes.

Drain Brussels sprouts and allow to cool, then slice each one in half.

Toss Brussel sprouts in a large mixing bowl with oil, parmesan cheese, crushed almonds, everything bagel seasoning, and salt.

If needed, use a wooden spoon to stir and make sure the Brussel sprouts are fully coated in seasoning.

Transfer the Brussels sprouts to the air fryer, and cook for 12 to 15 minutes at 375 or until golden for both sides.

Notes

Note: Nutrition information is a rough estimate only; actual values will vary based on the exact ingredients used and amount of recipe prepared.

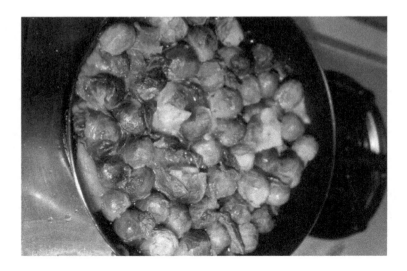

AIR FRYER VEGETABLE CHIPS

Preparation time 10 min.

Baking time 15 min.

Total time 25 min.

Ingredients

200 g parsnips

and or

200 g carrots

and or

2 pieces of beetroot

Spices as desired (e.g. sals, paprika powder, chilli, rosemary, etc.)

Preparation

Preheat the air fryer to 180 degrees for about 3 minutes.

Cut the vegetables, preferably with a vegetable slicer, into thin slices.

Since the different types of vegetables take different times in the air fryer to become crispy, you should prepare each one individually.

Parsnip chips: Place the thin parsnip slices in the basket of the hot air fryer and deep-fry them at 180 degrees for about 15 minutes.

Carrot chips: Place the thin carrot slices in the basket of the hot air fryer and deep-fry them at 180 degrees for about 20 minutes.

Beetroot chips: Place the thin beetroot slices in the basket of the hot air fryer and deep-fry them at 180 degrees for about 25 minutes.

To ensure that the vegetable chips are crispy on all sides, you should take the frying basket out of the hot air fryer about every 5 minutes and shake it well.

It is best to enjoy the vegetable chips straight away, as they will no longer be as crispy after a while.

After the vegetable chips are crispy, they can be refined with salt, paprika powder, chilli, rosemary or other spices, for example

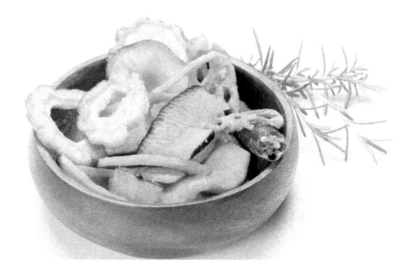

AIR FRYER CINNAMON QUARK BALLS

Preparation time: 5 Mins Cooking time: 30 Mins Total time: 35 Mins

ingredients

300 grams of curd

300 grams of flour 405

3 teaspoons of tartar baking powder

3 eggs

70 grams of sugar

½ teaspoon cinnamon

1 pinch of salt

a large pinch of ground vanilla

Mixture of sugar and cinnamon

Liquid butter

Preparation

Put the quark, salt, sugar, eggs, cinnamon, vanilla in the mixing bowl and mix for 35 seconds / speed 4.

Add baking powder and flour and add 2 minutes / kneading setting.

Either fry the quark balls in hot fat or use the Air fryer.

Preheat this to 180 degrees.

Use an ice cream scoop to put a large blob on the grill plate (please oil a little beforehand).

Bake the quark balls for 8 minutes at 180 degrees, then turn them over and another 3 minutes

With the amount of dough, you have to bake 3 times.

Then pour liquid butter on the quark balls and roll in the sugar-cinnamon mixture

Best to enjoy lukewarm.

Update: It is also possible in the oven: 180 degrees for 15 minutes!

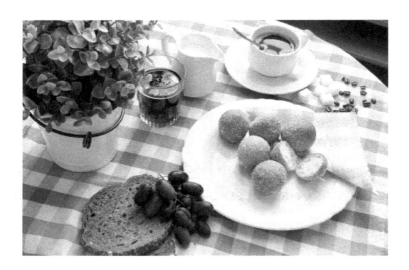

OVEN GREEN CURRY DRUMSTICKS

ingredient list

2 tablespoons (32 g)

green curry paste

1 tsp freshly grated ginger

2 tablespoons (8 g) fresh coriander

1/4 tsp Himalayan

salt

1/8 tsp Cayenne pepper

1/4 cup unsweetened full-fat yogurt or unsweetened non-dairy yogurt

2 tablespoons (30 ml) avocado oil

6th Chicken legs

Instructions

Mix the green curry paste, ginger, coriander, salt, cayenne pepper, yoghurt and oil in a food processor and stir until smooth. Pour the marinade into a large glass bowl and add the drumsticks;

throw to coat well. Cover the bowl and put it in the refrigerator for 3 hours or overnight.

Preheat the oven to 230 ° C, line a large baking sheet with foil and place a well-oiled grid in the pan. Place the marinated drumsticks on the prepared rack and put the pan in the oven for 45 minutes. Turn the drumsticks over halfway. At the end of the cooking time, turn the oven on roast and cook for another 3 to 5 minutes or until the drumsticks appear crispy. Take the pan out of the oven and let the drumsticks cool down a bit before serving. The drumsticks can be stored covered in the refrigerator for up to 3 days.

Substitutions: To make this recipe dairy-free or paleo, use unsweetened dairy-free yogurt. To make this recipe vegetarian, use paneer or tofu in place of chicken

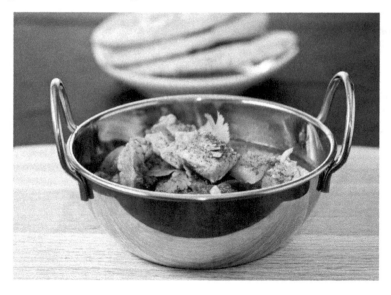

AIR FRYER VEGAN CHICKEN WINGS

preparation   10 Minutes

cooking time 50 Minutes

waiting period 50 Minutes

Servings   2 people

ingredient list

1 large cauliflower

100 G Chickpea flour or wheat flour

180 ml unsweetened soy or almond milk

60 ml water

2 Tl Garlic powder

1 1/2 Tl noble sweet paprika powder

salt

pepper

70 G Panko flour

250 ml Grill & Tex Mex Sauce

2 two spring onions

vegan aioli from Byodo for dipping

Sriracha sauce (optional)

Vegan chicken wings made from cauliflower

Instructions

Preheat the oven to 180 ° C.

In a large bowl, mix the flour, vegetable milk, water, garlic powder, paprika powder, salt and pepper.

Divide / cut the cauliflower into bite-sized florets. Dip the cauliflower florets in the flour mixture so that they are completely covered. The cauliflower wings also taste great when you add them to panko flour before baking. Panko flour is a breadcrumb from Japanese cuisine that gets really nice and crispy. Line a baking sheet with parchment paper and distribute the cauliflower florets evenly on it. Do not lay on top of each other. Bake for 25 minutes.

Take the cauliflower out of the oven after 25 minutes and dip it in the Tex-Mex sauce or, alternatively, spread it evenly over the cauliflower florets. If you want the vegan cauliflower wings a little hotter, you can spread a little Sriracha sauce over them. Bake again for 25 minutes.

Cut the spring onions into rings and spread over the vegan cauliflower chicken wings. Serve with the vegan aioli.

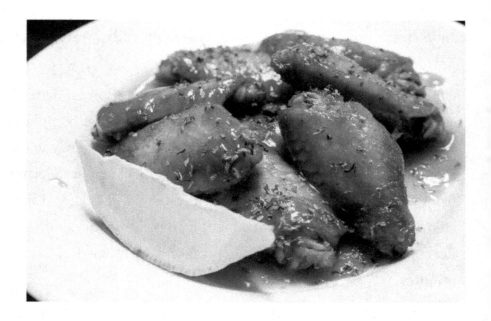

AIR FRYER BROCCOLI

Preparation time: 10 min

Preparation time: 30 min

Total time: 40 min

Servings: 10

Ingredients

1 broccoli

4 eggs

100 gr almond flour

1/2 tsp sea salt

2 pinches of black pepper

optional: dried herbs for it

Instructions

Preheat the oven to 175°C

Chop the broccoli into rice with the pulse function of your food processor. You can also use a food chopper or chop the broccoli by hand.

Beat the eggs in a mixing bowl. Add the broccoli rice, almond flour, sea salt and black pepper. Mix into a thick dough

Spoon the dough onto a baking tray covered with parchment paper. Use a spatula to spread the dough until it is about 1/2 inch thick.

Bake for 30 minutes or more until golden brown

Let it cool for at least 10 minutes. Turnover and remove the parchment paper. Cut it into square pieces and keep it in a large glass jar in the refrigerator

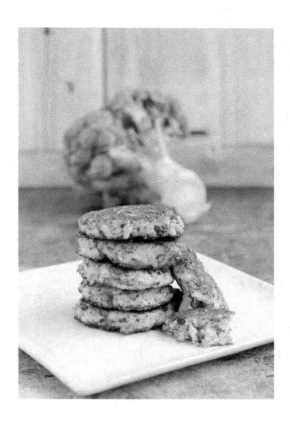

AIR FRYER BLISSFUL SALMON

Ingredients

For the fish (per person):

1 slice of (defrosted) salmon - wild salmon because of the healthy fats, MSC quality mark because of the responsible fishing

pepper and salt or fish seasoning, to taste

2-3 slices of bacon

1 tbsp pesto

1-2 sprigs of thyme (preferably lemon thyme)

20 g feta

For with it (per person):

2 snack tomatoes

pepper, salt, 1 basil leaf

1 tsp pine nuts

To step

Per person:

Sprinkle the salmon steak on both sides with salt and pepper or with fish herbs. Massage the herbs in a little with your hand.

Place the bacon slices on a plate. For the largest salmon steak, I used 3 slices, for the rest 2 was sufficient.

Spread half of the pesto on the bottom of the salmon steak and then place it with the pesto side on the bacon. The salmon has been turned over for the photo.

Then spread the rest of the pesto on top. Crumble the feta over it. Remove the leaves from the thyme and sprinkle them over the feta.

Wrap the bacon around the salmon.

Finishing and baking:

Preheat the Air fryer to 180 degrees Celsius.

Halve the snack tomatoes. This is easiest with a serrated / tomato knife. It is easy if they stay together on the side, then they do not wobble. Cut the basil leaves into strips. Sprinkle salt and pepper and the basil strips over the tomatoes and place them between the salmon steaks.

Sprinkle the pine nuts over the dish.

Place the dish in the Airfyrer for about 15 minutes, or until the bacon is nice and crispy. And then... feast!

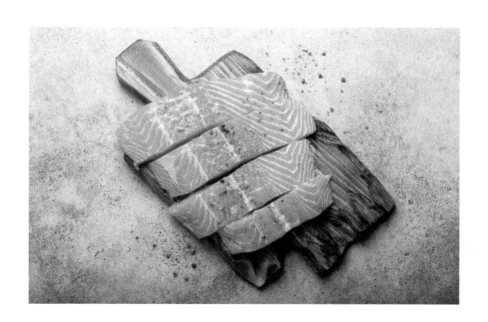

AIR FRYER BROCCOLI

Prep Time: 2 minutes

Cook Time: 8 minutes

0 minutes

Total Time: 10 minutes

Servings: 2 servings

Ingredients

3-4 cups broccoli florets

2 tablespoons olive oil

1/4 teaspoon garlic powder

1/4 teaspoon salt

1/4 teaspoon pepper

Instructions

Add broccoli, olive oil, garlic powder, salt & pepper to a large bowl and toss to combine.

Transfer to air fryer and set to 375F for 8 minutes. Shake halfway through.

Once the timer goes off, remove and serve immediately.

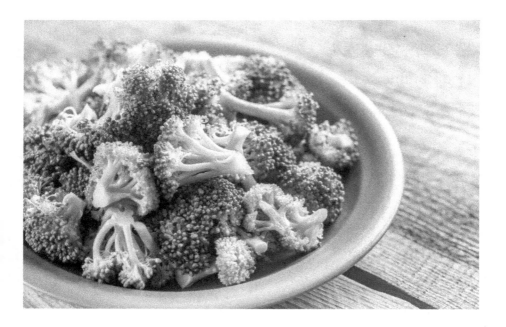

AIR FRYER CAULIFLOWER CROQUETTES!

Ingredients

6 croquettes

1.2 khd per croquette

300 g of cauliflower

75 g parmesan cheese

1 egg

1/2 tsp paprika

2 sprigs of chopped coriander

pepper

50 g bacon

15 g parmesan cheese

Preparation method:

Cut the cauliflower into florets and cook them al dente. Puree the cauliflower and squeeze the excess moisture from the cauliflower puree with a kitchen towel.

Mix the cauliflower puree with the parmesan cheese, egg, paprika, coriander and pepper and make 6 croquettes.

Chop the bacon with a food processor and add the parmesan cheese.

(if you don't like bacon, you can also use only parmesan cheese or finely ground low-carb crackers)

Put the croquettes through the finely ground bacon and parmesan cheese and put them in the airfryer at 180c for 10 minutes.

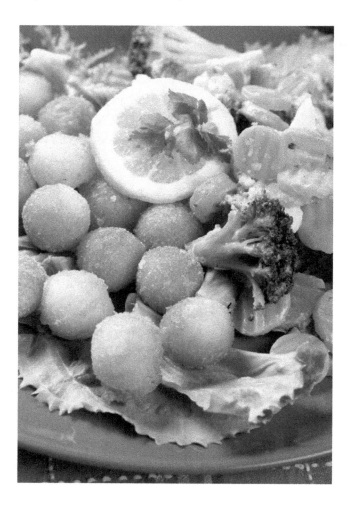

AIR FRYER CRISPY TOFU

Prep: 30 minutes Cook: 15 minutes Total: 45 minutes servings: 4

Ingredients

1 16-oz block extra-firm tofu 453 g

2 Tbsp soy sauce 30 mL

1 Tbsp toasted sesame oil* 15 mL

1 Tbsp olive oil 15 mL

1 clove garlic minced

Instructions

Press: Press tofu for at least 15 minutes, using either a or by setting a heavy pan on top of it, letting the moisture drain. When finished, cut tofu into bite-sized blocks and transfer to a bowl.

Flavor: Combine all remaining ingredients in a small bowl. Drizzle over tofu and toss to coat. Let tofu marinate for an additional 15 minutes.

Air Fry: Preheat your air fryer to 375 degrees F (190 C). Add tofu blocks to your air fryer basket in a single layer. Cook for 10 to 15 minutes, shaking the pan occasionally to promote even cooking.

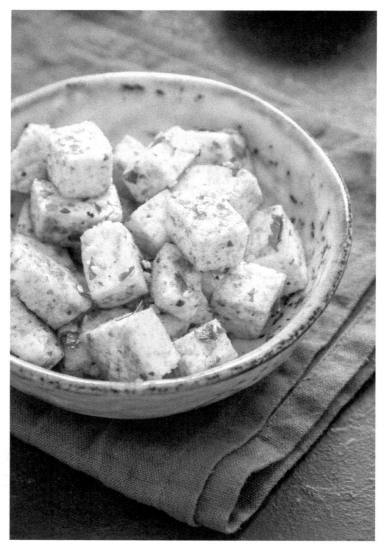

AIR FRYER BEEF KOFTA KABAB

Prep Time: 10 minutes Cook Time: 10 minutes Total Time: 20 minutes servings: 4

Ingredients

1 tablespoon (1 tablespoon) Oil

1 pound (453.59 g) Lean Ground Beef

¼ cup (15 g) Chopped Parsley

1 tablespoon (1 tablespoon) Minced Garlic

2 tablespoons (2 tablespoons) kofta kabab spice mix

1 teaspoon (1 teaspoon) Kosher Salt

Instructions

Using a stand mixer, blend together all ingredients. If you have time, let the mixture sit in the fridge for 30 minutes. You can also mix it up and set aside for a day or two until you're ready to make the kababs

Although I tried this with and without skewers, it really makes no difference to the final product. Since it's a lot easier to simply shape the kababs by hand, divide the meat into four and make four long sausage shapes (or Pokémon shape or whatever you want).

Place the kababs in your air fryer and cook at 370F for 10 minutes.

Check with a meat thermometer to ensure that the kababs have an internal temperature of 145F.

Sprinkle with additional parsley for garnishing and serve with tzatziki, a cucumber tomato salad, and pita bread.

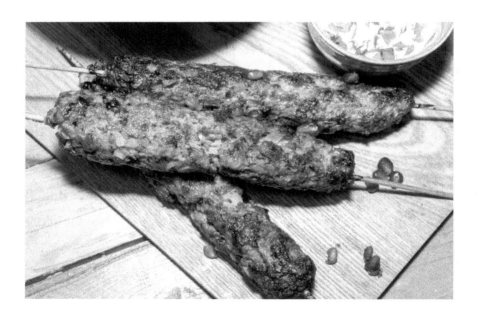

AIRFRYER HEALTHY SANDWICH

Ingredients

4 slices of white floor bread

4 slices of Gouda young matured

2 slices of roasted ham

15 g unsalted butter in the tub

Instructions

Preheat the airfryer to 180 ° C. Cover a slice of bread successively with a slice of cheese, slice of ham and another slice of cheese. Cover with a slice of bread. Make another sandwich like this.

Spread the outside of the sandwich with half the butter. Bake 1 sandwich in the airfryer for 5 minutes until golden brown. Turn halfway through. Bake another sandwich in this way.

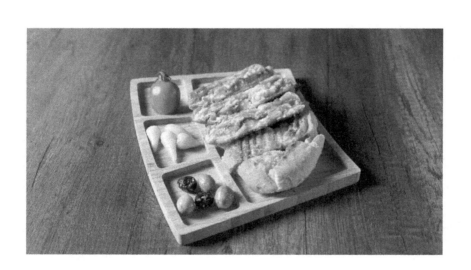

VEGETABLE PAPRIKA CHIPS

Servings 5,

Cooking time: 15-20 minutes

Ingredients

1 small parsnip

3 carrots (suggestion: take three different colored carrots)

¼ celeriac

¼ swede

1 tablespoon of paprika

½ teaspoon of garlic powder

½ teaspoon chili powder

Pinch of salt

3 eggs

1 tablespoon of mustard

100 grams of Panko

250ml Greek yogurt 0%

2 cloves of garlic

3 tablespoons of freshly chopped chives

Instructions

Bring a pan with water and some salt to the boil. Wash all vegetables and then peel them. Cut thick fries and blanch them briefly. Rinse with cold water and drain well.

Beat the eggs with the spices and mix it all the way through the sliced vegetable fries. Now sprinkle the panko over the wet fries and mix well with your hands.

Cover the bottom of the basket with the chips, but make sure it is not overfilled. Bake the fries for 15 to 20 minutes at 180 degrees. Shake them twice in between.

Make the yogurt sauce while baking. Cut the chives and squeeze the garlic cloves and mix them with the yogurt. Season with salt and pepper from the mill. Then serve the fries with the yoghurt sauce

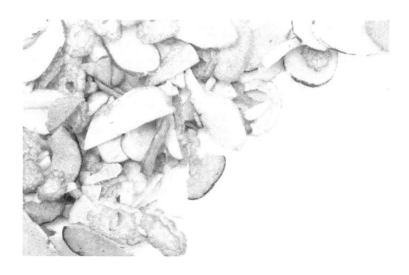

ZUCCHINI AND CHEESE BREAD

Ingredients

1 tbsp olive oil

1 onion

2 cloves of garlic

100 gr ham

450 g zucchini

200 gr feta

200 gr ricotta

40 gr grated old cheese

6 sprigs of thyme

60 gr green olives without stone

6 eggs

150 g spelled bread flour (or regular flour, that is also possible)

Instructions

Preheat the oven to 180 degrees (electric) or 160 degrees (hot air). Grease a 20x30cm baking pan with butter. And then cover with baking paper.

Finely chop the onion and garlic, put the olive oil in a frying pan and fry the onion and garlic on low heat for 3-5 minutes until golden brown.

Grate the zucchini. Chop the olives roughly and crumble the feta. Put everything in a large bowl and add the ricotta and grated old cheese. Spoon the onion and garlic into the mixture. Remove the leaves from the thyme sprigs and add. Cut the ham into strips and add some salt to the mixture.

Stir the eggs, add the flour and stir until it becomes a smooth mixture. Add to the zucchini mix and stir well.

Spoon the mixture into the baking tin and smooth the top. Bake for 40-50 minutes or until the top is golden brown. Prick the courgetti bread with a wooden skewer to see if the bread is cooked properly. The skewer must come out of the bread dry. If not, put it back in the oven. Cut the bread into 10 pieces.

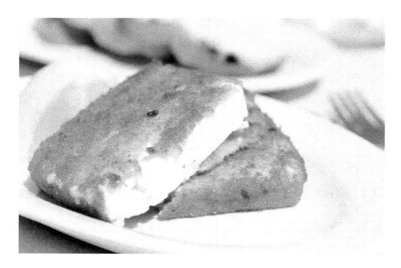

LOW CARB PARMESAN BREAD

Ingredients

Based on 2 people

Parmesan grated

5 tbsp

almond flour

3 tbsp

baking powder

½ tsp

melted butter

1 tbsp

1 egg

Instructions

Mix all dry ingredients in a bowl.

Add egg and butter and mix all ingredients.

Divide the dough between a few buttered coffee cups or in a muffin tin.

You can quickly prepare this in the microwave. Then they are ready in 3 to 5 minutes

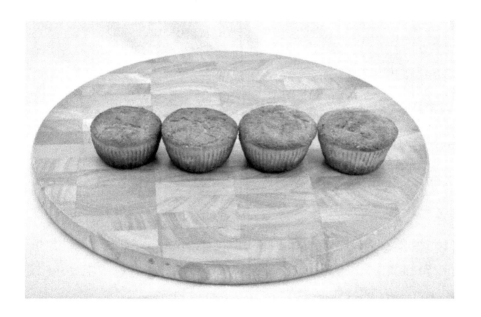

AIRFRYER CINNAMON CARROT CAKE

Ingredients

140 g Soft brown sugar

2 eggs, beaten

140 g butter

1 orange, zest & juice

200 g self-raising flour

1 tsp ground cinnamon

175 g grated carrot, (approx. 2 medium carrots)

60 g sultana

Instructions

Preheat air fryer to 160C.

In a bowl, cream together the butter and sugar.

Slowly add the beaten eggs.

Fold in the flour, a little bit at a time, mixing it as you go. Add the orange juice and zest, grated carrots and sultanas. Gently mix all the ingredients together.

Grease the baking tin and pour the mixture in.

Place baking tin in the air fryer basket and cook for 30 minutes. Check and see if the cake has cooked - use a cocktail stick or metal skewer to poke in the middle. If it comes out wet then cook it for a little longer.

Remove the baking tin from the airfryer basket and allow to cool for 10 minutes before removing from the basket.

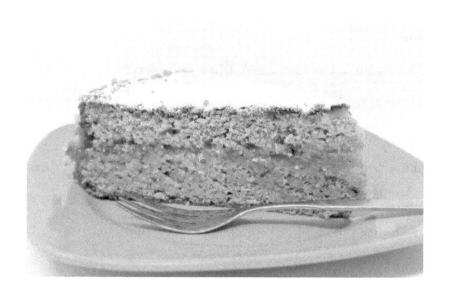

AIR FRYER ALMOND CHICKEN

Prep time: 10 mins

Ingredients

Marinade

2 lbs. chicken breast tenders, cut into small pieces

2 cups almond milk

1 tsp salt

½ tsp black pepper

½ ground paprika

Dry Ingredients

3 cups flour

3 tsp salt

2 tsp black pepper

2 tsp paprika

oil spray

Instructions

In a large Ziplock bag, add the chicken and all of the marinade ingredients. Marinate in the refrigerator for at least 2 hours, up to 6 hours.

In a large shallow bowl, add all of the dry ingredients.

After marinating, place chicken and marinade into a large bowl. Working in small batches, dredge chicken chunks into dry ingredients, shake off excess flour, dunk again briefly into the marinade, then dredge for a second time in the dry ingredients, fully coating each piece of chicken. Be sure to gently shake off excess flour mixture.

Spray olive oil onto the bottom and sides of the inside of the air fryer vessel. Place breaded chicken in an even layer; set aside the rest of the chicken. Give the tops of the chicken in the air fryer vessel a quick spray with olive oil, then place into the air fryer.

Air fry at 370°F for 10 minutes. Halfway through this cooking time (at 5 minutes), open the air fryer and shake the basket. If using a tray-style air fryer, use tongs to turn chicken pieces over. Spray tops of chicken with cooking spray, then resume air frying for the remaining 5 minutes.

NOTE: depending on the size and amount of chicken, you may need to allow yours to cook in the air fryer for 2-3 minutes more.

Remove from the air fryer, and repeat steps until you're finished with all of the chicken (usually 3 to 4 batches for me; it may be more or less for you, depending on your air fryer and also how you cut your chicken pieces).

Serve immediately with your favorite dipping sauces. Place any extra chicken into freezer-safe plastic bags and freeze for up to 3 months.

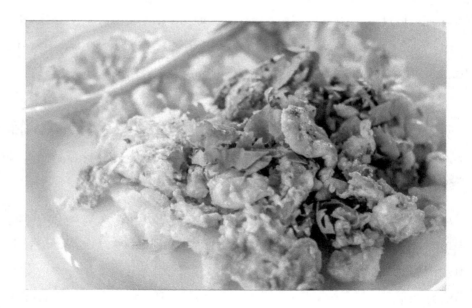

DUCK BREAST SAUCE

Preparation Time: 10 minutes Cooking Time: 32 minutes

Servings: 2

Ingredients

Two duck breasts

1 tbsp. butter

1-star anise

1 tbsp. olive oil

One shallot

9 oz. red plumps

2 tbsp. sugar

2 tbsp. red wine

1 cup beef stock

Directions:

Heat a pan over medium heat with the olive oil, add shallot, stir and cook for 5 minutes,

Add sugar and plums, stir and cook until sugar dissolves.

Add stock and wine, stir, cook for 15 minutes, take off the heat and keep warm for now.

Score duck breasts, season with salt and pepper, rub with melted butter, transfer to a heatproof dish that fits your air fryer, add star anise and plum sauce, introduce in your air fryer and cook at 360 degrees F for 12 minutes.

Divide everything among plates and serve.

TASTY CRISPY CHICKEN BREASTS

Preparation Time: 15 minutes Cooking Time: 12 minutes
Servings: 6

Ingredients:

1 cup panko breadcrumbs

½ cup Parmesan cheese, grated

¼ cup fresh rosemary, minced

¼ tsp. cayenne pepper

Salt and ground black pepper, as required

6 (4-ounce) boneless, skinless chicken breasts

3 tbsps. olive oil

Olive oil cooking spray

Directions:

In a shallow dish, add the breadcrumbs, Parmesan cheese, rosemary, cayenne pepper, salt, and black pepper and mix well.

Rub the chicken breasts with oil and then coat with the breadcrumbs mixture evenly.

Arrange the chicken breasts onto the steak tray and spray with cooking spray.

Select "Air Fry" of Air Fryer Oven and then adjust the temperature to 350 degrees F.

Set the timer for 12 minutes and press "Start/Stop" to begin cooking.

When the unit beeps to show that it is preheated, insert the steak tray in the Air fryer Oven.

Flip the chicken breasts once halfway through.

If the cooking time is complete, remove the chicken breasts from Air fryer Oven and serve hot.

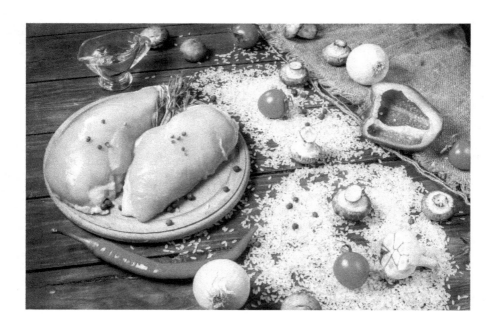

PAPRIKA CHICKEN TENDERS

Preparation Time: 5 minutes Cooking Time: 12 minutes
Servings: 4

Ingredients:

1 pound (454 g) chicken tenders

1 tsp. kosher salt

1 tsp. black pepper

½ tsp. smoked paprika

¼ cup coarse mustard

2tbsps. honey

1 cup finely crushed pecans

Directions:

Press Start/Cancel. Preheat the air fryer oven, set the temperature to 350°F (177°C).

Place the chicken in a large bowl. Sprinkle with salt, pepper, and paprika. Toss until the spices are mixed with the chicken. Add the mustard and honey and toss until the chicken is coated.

Place the pecans on a plate. Roll the chicken into the pecans until both sides are coated, dealing with one piece of chicken at a time. Lightly brush off any loose pecans. Place the chicken in the fry basket. Insert at a low position.

Select Bake, Convection, and set time to 12 minutes or until the chicken be cooked through and the pecans are golden brown.

Serve warm.

CHICKEN THIGHS WITH PEANUTS

Preparation Time: 10 minutes Cooking Time: 20 minutes
Servings: 6

Ingredients:

½ cup unsweetened full-fat
coconut milk

2 tbsps. yellow curry paste

1 tbsp. minced fresh ginger

1 tbsp. minced garlic

1 tsp. kosher salt

1 pound or (454 g) boneless,
skinless chicken thighs,
halved crosswise

2 tbsps. chopped peanuts

Directions:

In a large bowl, stir together the coconut milk, curry paste, ginger, garlic, and salt until well blended. Add the chicken; toss well to coat. Marinate for 30 minutes and cover or refrigerate for up to 24 hours.

Press Start/Cancel. Preheat the air fryer oven to 375°F (191°C).

Place the chicken (along with marinade) in a baking pan. Place the pan in the fry basket. Insert at a low position.

Select Bake, Convection, and set time to 20 minutes, turning the chicken halfway through the cooking time. Use a meat thermometer to ensure the chicken has reached an internal temperature of 165°F (74°C).

Sprinkle with the chopped peanuts over the chicken and serve.

SIMPLE CHICKEN THIGHS

Preparation Time: 10 minutes Cooking Time: 35 minutes Servings: 6

Ingredients

Six chicken thighs

2 tsp. poultry seasoning

2 tbsp. olive oil

Pepper

Salt

Directions

Insert wire rack in rack position 6. Select bake, set temperature 390 f, timer for 40 minutes. Press start to preheat the oven.

Brush chicken with oil and rub with poultry seasoning, pepper, and salt.

Arrange chicken on roasting pan and bake for 35-40 minutes or until internal temperature reaches 165 f.

Serve and enjoy. Nutrition: Calories319 kcal

BBQ CHICKEN WINGS

Preparation Time: 10 minutes Cooking Time: 55 minutes
Servings: 8

Ingredients

32 chicken wings

1 1/2 cups BBQ sauce

1/4 cup olive oil

Pepper

Salt

Directions

Line baking sheet using parchment paper and set aside.

Insert wire rack in rack position 6. Select bake, set temperature 375 f, timer for 55 minutes. Press start to preheat the oven.

In a mixing bowl, toss chicken wings with olive oil, pepper, and salt.

Arrange chicken wings on a baking sheet and bake for 50 minutes.

Toss chicken wings with BBQ sauce and bake for 5 minutes more.

Serve and enjoy

ORANGE JUICE MARINATED STEAK

Preparation Time: 6 minutes Cooking Time: 60 minutes

Servings: 4

Ingredients

¼ cup orange juice

1 tsp. ground cumin

2 pounds skirt steak, trimmed from excess fat

2 tbsps. lime juice

2 tbsps. olive oil

Four cloves of garlic, minced

Salt and pepper to taste

Directions:

Put all ingredients in a mixing bowl and allow to marinate in the fridge for at least 2 hours

Preheat the air fryer oven to 390°F.

Place the grill pan accessory in the air fryer.

Grill for 15 minutes per batch and flip the beef every 8 minutes for even grilling.

Meanwhile, pour the marinade on a saucepan and allow to simmer for 10 minutes or until the sauce thickens.

Slice the beef and pour over the sauce.

Conclusion

We have come to the conclusion of this journey into the taste of fried food but in a healthy way. If you picked up this book I imagine you already have an air fryer, but if not, I'm sure you'll soon have this marvel in your kitchen. Having an air fryer in your home is an added value that is becoming more and more popular.

Now you have the ideas for cooking, all that's left to do is start putting them into practice.

Enjoy!!!

Thank you for reading this cookbook

Violet H. Scott

CPSIA information can be obtained
at www.ICGtesting.com
Printed in the USA
BVHW060723050521
606421BV00003B/563

9 781802 671223